Instructional Methods in Emergency Services

Second Edition

William D. McClincy
EMS Program Specialist
EMMCO West, Inc.
Meadville, Pennsylvania

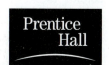

Prentice
Hall

Upper Saddle River, New Jersey 07458

Library of Congress Cataloging-in-Publication Data

McClincy, William D.

    Instructional methods in emergency services / William D. McClincy.—2nd ed.

      p.   cm.

    Includes index.

    ISBN 0-13-033127-9

    1. Emergency medical services—Study and teaching.   2. Rescue work—Study and teaching.   3. Fire extinction—Study and teaching.   I. Title.

RA645.5 .M39 2002

616.02′5′0715—dc21

2001058014

Publisher: *Julie Levin Alexander*
Assistant to Publisher: *Regina Bruno*
Senior Acquisitions Editor: *Katrin Beacom*
Editorial Assistant: *Kierra Kashickey*
Senior Marketing Manager: *Tiffany Price*
Product Information Manager: *Rachelle Triano*
Director of Production and Manufacturing: *Bruce Johnson*
Managing Production Editor: *Patrick Walsh*
Manufacturing Buyer: *Pat Brown*
Production Liaison: *Julie Li*
Production Editor: *Lori Johnson*
Media Development Editor: *Sarah Hayday*
Manager of Media Production: *Amy Peltier*
New Media Project Manager: *Stephen J. Hartner*
Creative Director: *Cheryl Asherman*
Cover Design Coordinator: *Maria Guglielmo*
Cover Designer: *Gary J. Sella*
Composition: *BookMasters, Inc.*
Printing and Binding: *Courier Westford*

Pearson Education LTD.
Pearson Education Australia PTY, Limited
Pearson Education Singapore, Pte. Ltd
Pearson Education North Asia Ltd
Pearson Education Canada, Ltd.
Pearson Educación de Mexico, S.A. de C.V.
Pearson Education—Japan
Pearson Education Malaysia, Pte. Ltd
Pearson Education, Upper Saddle River, New Jersey

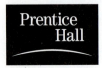

10 9 8 7 6 5 4 3 2 1

ISBN 0-13-033127-9

This book is dedicated to my wife Valerie, my son Everett, and my daughter Jessica. Their love and support are unending and are my main motivators in my life.

Contents

Foreword

Having spent almost 20 years in the field of emergency services education, I have seen many books come across my desk, but what a welcome relief to have the opportunity to experience *Instructional Methods in Emergency Services*.

The field of emergency services education has needed for years a concise, well-written, but most importantly, practical, hands-on approach to demonstrating the complexities of the education process, coupled with the challenging journey of teaching emergency service personnel. I have grown tired of seeing volumes on book racks that claim to teach educational practices of hands-on methodology, and of course, the use of the latest in instructional modalities including CD-ROM and the internet. Many authors claim instant success by using their products in teaching adult students.

Just when I'd despaired of finding an objective, informative, and interesting text, what should arrive but *Instructional Methods in Emergency Services*—what a treat! I thoroughly enjoy this textbook because it is easy to understand, has lots of illustrations, and utilizes many charts, graphs, and references for easy comprehension.

Perhaps one of the reasons *Instructional Methods in Emergency Services* is so objective and practical is that it is written by an emergency service educator and practitioner who believes in what he "preaches" and presents his classroom experience in a dynamic, enjoyable manner.

Every textbook on the topic of education has its own particular slant or emphasis, and this one is no exception. Bill McClincy has developed his own perception of how to effectively teach adults based upon years of experience in a variety of classroom and nonclassroom teaching/training/facilitating activities. The contents are not intended to be a way to teach adults, but the author's perspective is to show emergency services educators, new or experienced, how to examine the strategies available for use in teaching adults—sort of a "tool box" approach.

The author acknowledges the respective strengths and limitations of educational strategies as applied to emergency services and provides suggestions for their effective use in various teaching/learning situations.

Whether you are new to the field or an old-timer, you will have one happy adventure!

Everitt F. Binns, Ph.D.
Executive Director
Eastern Pennsylvania Emergency Medical Services Council

Preface

This is the second edition of *Instructional Methods in Emergency Services.* The first edition was a groundbreaking textbook. Until its publication, few textbooks had been written that discussed the nuances of emergency service instruction. Seasoned and new instructors will find interactive and exciting information within this edition.

Instructional Methods in Emergency Services, Second Edition builds upon the principles and concepts identified in the first edition. This second edition incorporates the latest educational trends and information needed to create innovative and motivational presentations.

A unique facet of the second edition is its integrated computer-based instruction and Internet applications. Information, especially digital, cannot be explained in a printed form, rather it needs to be seen and experienced. The CD-ROM, included with the second edition, incorporates these qualities and allows digital forms of information to be experienced. Internet links, computerized instruction programs, and the use of PowerPoint applications are some of the applications included on the CD-ROM.

Successful and respected educators strive for excellence in their presentations. Instructors and students bring enriched experiences to the classroom. Instructors need to know their limitations in order to be able to create instructional programs that foster behavioral changes in their students. *Instructional Methods in Emergency Services, Second Edition* provides instructors with tools needed to create, improve, augment, and enrich their presentations. Instructors blend their personalities, knowledge, and experience with these tools to create effective presentations.

Quality education starts and ends with competent and knowledgeable instruction. Today's students demand that educational programs be informative and challenging. *Instructional Methods in Emergency Services, Second Edition* and its CD-ROM are valuable resources for instructors to use throughout their years of instructional experience.

This textbook can be used as a primary text in initial instructor training programs or as a resource for seasoned instructors. Enjoy both the textbook and CD-ROM as you develop your instructional presentations.

Acknowledgments

A textbook is the culmination of a lot of work by a lot of people. Without the support, guidance, assistance, and commitment of the following people, this second edition would not have been possible:

To Val, Everett, and Jessica for allowing me the time to work on this revision.

A special thanks to all the people at Brady/Prentice Hall Health Publishing. Katrin Beacom, Judy Streger, Greg Vis, Sarah Hayday, and Tiffany Price have been great assets throughout this revision process. Thanks for allowing me the opportunity to share my insights and experience with other instructors and colleagues.

I must thank two special individuals who have been instrumental in this textbook revision, Richard Hernan and Everitt Binns. Rick, your legal expertise and insights have greatly enhanced the revised legal aspects chapter. Ev, both as a friend and a colleague, your insights have kept my focus on what's important in my life and are also reflected throughout this revision.

Many of the photos used in the original textbook and in this revision are courtesy of Richard Gibbons, Jr. He is not only a great photographer, but is a dynamic leader and team builder. I am honored to work with him and all my other coworkers at EMMCO West.

Finally, I want to acknowledge and thank the students with whom I have been able to share my experience. Every instructor program I have conducted has been a unique and enlightening experience. No one program has ever been the same. My experience with students taking an instructor trainer program is that they aspire to share their experiences with others. This textbook helps instructors learn who they are, so they can become successful and respected educators.

Chapter 1

Introduction

➤ **OBJECTIVES**

- Define the term *methodology*.
- Provide an overview of each of the chapters discussed within the book.
- Identify how each of the chapters is interlinked with one another.
- Introduce multimedia adjuncts and learning activities contained on the interactive CD-ROM.
- Review basic principles of computers, hardware/software, and the Internet.
- Identify the illustrations from the Baker Street Group.
- Identify the variety of illustrations, charts, and photographs found throughout the book.
- Review the format that is contained in each chapter.
- Identify suggested uses of the book's content.

. . . a vehicle accident at the intersection of Maple and Walnut Streets . . . EMS, Fire, and Rescue respond . . . confirmed entrapment . . . police on scene advise two critical injuries . . . additional units requested . . .

A typical emergency response to which emergency medical service (EMS), fire, and rescue personnel respond on a daily basis. The street address changes, the number of patients and cars involved changes, and the crews that respond to the accident scene change—but what does not change is the expected quality of care and services provided by these emergency personnel. Every incident requires superior performance from emergency personnel.

Where do emergency personnel attain the knowledge to handle these daily events? The answer is from training programs. Information is passed on from qualified instructors. Information is presented in a way that is informative yet interesting and motivating. Emergency personnel are expected to deliver quality care and services at the scene of an emergency. This can happen only if they have had quality instruction during their training programs.

What is "quality" training? How does an instructor design a presentation that will be informative, interesting, and motivating? Part of the answer is found in the term *methodology. Methodology* is defined by *Webster's* as

The system of methods as in any particular science..[1]

---

[1]*From Webster's New World™ College Dictionary, 4th Edition.* Copyright © 2000, 1999 by Hungry Minds, Inc. All rights reserved. Reproduced here by permission of the publisher.

When teaching emergency personnel, an instructor uses all three of these elements. The instructor puts together a lesson that is interesting and involves the students in the learning process.

To make a presentation come alive is a challenge for the instructor. Any instructor can make a lesson presentation. But only those who create an educational experience—that is, make the dullest of subjects interesting—become quality instructors.

For quality education to occur, the starting point is with the instructor. If the instructor cannot make quality presentations, the overall learning experience is affected:

$$\text{Quality instruction} = \text{Quality education}$$

Together, they determine the quality of care or services provided in the field.

This book provides the principles, practices, and procedures to become a quality instructor. Students, instructors, teaching techniques, facilities, equipment, administration, subject material, plus countless other factors influence the educational environment. To be a successful instructor, an instructor must be able to understand how these factors influence a presentation. Successful instructors are able to use these factors to their advantage and to create a positive learning experience.

Chapter Style

The chapters are arranged in an order that follows the creation of a lesson plan. The preparation of a lesson is reviewed in Chapters 2, 3, 4, 5, 6, and 7. In Chapters 8 and 9, the actual methods of instruction are discussed. Chapters 10, 11, 12, and 13 identify the course evaluation process and look at the different enhancements used in training programs. Finally, Chapters 14 and 15 deal with legal issues and administrative issues that affect the operation of a course and/or training institute.

Where it has been possible, complex educational terms have been replaced with commonly used words: Being an instructor does not mean that you need to use $10 words when penny phrases will have the same effect. So when reading this book, you will see penny phrases instead of $10 terms.

Interlinking and Interrelating Among Chapters

Behavioral objectives are important in creating and conducting an entire lesson presentation. In almost every chapter, there are details involving behavioral objectives. Even though Chapter 5, "Behavioral Objectives, Lesson Plans, and Curriculum," tells how to write and use behavioral objectives, other chapters provide information on how to use the behavioral objectives. Chapter 6 uses objectives to identify audiovisual (AV) aids. Chapter 8 uses behavioral objectives to define the type of teaching approaches used to instruct a course. Chapter 9 identifies how behavioral objectives affect the conduction of a skill presentation. Chapter 10 uses the objectives to write examination questions and determine a question's difficulty. Reading Chapter 5 is just the starting point for understanding behavioral objectives.

Other chapters show how behavioral objectives impact the specific topics that are being discussed. There is a natural interrelationship between objectives and the other material being discussed in this book. Behavioral objectives are the most frequently interrelated subject, but they are not the only one. Realism, AV aids, and evaluation topics are also found in different chapters, aside from their own specific chapters. So when you are reading about a topic, such as behavioral objectives, look for additional information in other related chapters.

It is a pleasure to introduce "Vic and Vern" (see Figure 1-1). The duo will appear in various sketches throughout the book. The motto for Vic and Vern is, "Vic and Vern, here to help you learn." Vic and Vern are based on actual characters from the music/comedy group "The Dysrhythmics"; the sketches are courtesy of the Baker Street Group.

It's okay to laugh when you see one of the sketches, but realize that when you see the "Mr. War Stories" sketch, there is a message that Vic and Vern want you to recognize about teaching emergency service programs.

Photographs, Sidebars, Internet, CD-ROM

Vic and Vern's sketches are humorous and informative, but additional information can be gained from photographs, graphs, sidebars, Internet addresses, and the interactive CD-ROM.

Many of the photographs are from actual incidents or are from training programs. Specific sections of the book, for example, the realism photographs, were created just for this textbook. Photographs provide a unique message to supplement the written material. The phrase, "a picture is worth a thousand words," is one of the main reasons why photographs are used both in educational training programs and why they are used in this book.

When detailed information has been discussed, charts and diagrams have been included to supplement the written material. These diagrams provide clarity to the material that is being discussed. Included are pie charts, normal curves, mathematical formulas, and a variety of training program scenarios.

Internet sites included in this textbook, at the time of publishing, are considered valid Internet addresses. Due to the dynamics of the Internet, sites change their Internet addresses.

Special material has been included in sidebars. Included next to the main text, there are special information boxes that tell related stories about the topic being discussed. Not every chapter has them, but when you find one of these sidebars, stop and read the information.

Internet access is a part of many emergency service classrooms. More and more computer interactive programs are being introduced on almost a daily basis. Virtual classrooms, found on the World Wide Web (WWW), are replacing traditional four-wall classrooms. Initial and continuing education courses can be accessed upon demand. The Internet is a vital resource for instructors. Instructors can access countless resources to develop their lesson presentations and then take their students on virtual trips to a variety of interactive programs. Throughout this textbook, you will find "www links" to online instruction resource sites, i.e. www.bradybooks.com. Chapter 12 further explains the Internet and identifies specific applications and sites.

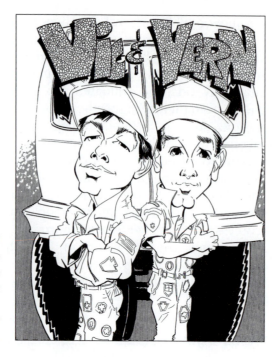

Figure 1-1
Featured are the
characters from the
Dysrhythmics, Vic
and Vern.
Courtesy of the Baker
Street Group, Inc.

Included with this textbook, you will find a CD-ROM. This CD contains
a variety of information, resources, simulations, PowerPoint presentations,
and chapter activities. Insert the CD-ROM into your computer. Click on the
CD-ROM drive; the CD-ROM is a self-loading CD. Follow the directions on
the main menu screen and enjoy your virtual learning experience.

Chapter Format

Just like a lesson plan, this book is based on the objectives. The objectives
have been formed from various instructional curriculums and reference
materials. If you want to know the contents of a chapter, just look at the
objectives.

Each chapter is concluded with a summary of the chapter's material. Many of the chapters are quite lengthy. The chapter summary puts
the chapter's main points into a series of condensed paragraphs. If you
want the gist of a chapter, read the introduction and the chapter summary. This will give you a good idea of what is being discussed within
the chapter.

Depending on the chapter, you may need to do a little homework! Included within specific chapters or located on the CD-ROM are various interactive activities. These activities can be used as homework assignments,
for small group discussions, or as enrichments to the chapter material.

With the exception of this chapter, the remaining chapters are written from a colleague's perspective. In this introduction chapter, the word *you* often is used. You is being used to focus your attention on the aspects of the book that are important to recognize. Anyone using this book is considered a colleague, a fellow instructor.

Each chapter begins with the objectives, an introduction, a main text, the chapter summary, and interactive learning activities. The main text reflects the historical, traditional, present-day, and future trends of emergency service training programs.

An Overview of the Book

So what is this book about? What material does it cover? Use this section as a quick reference to what a chapter is about.

CHAPTER 2, ADULT LEARNERS AND THEIR CHARACTERISTICS

In most emergency service training programs, the majority of students fall into the adult learner category. Adult learners are characteristically self-motivated individuals who attend programs to better themselves. Adult learners need more hands-on training and fewer lecture-based activities. Knowing how adult learners learn and retain information is crucial. These adult learning characteristics are reviewed and explored.

Instructors need to design a lesson plan around the students. A student with little or no emergency service background, compared to a student who is enrolled in a refresher or continuing education course, will affect how instructors write and present their lesson material. A critical element facing instructors is the diversity of students within a class. There will likely be a mixture of students with varied educational backgrounds. You may have advanced level students who will be bored by basic lesson material, while at the same time there will be new students who are excited by the same material. If instructors can identify their classes' mix, a variety of classroom activities can be planned for the educational levels of the students.

CHAPTER 3, INSTRUCTORS AND THEIR CHARACTERISTICS

Anyone can design a lesson plan, but it takes an instructor to present the material. Instructors must be able to motivate their students. For a presentation to come alive takes qualities unique to an instructor. There are artistic skills, referred to as the "art of the little things," that instructors use to make presentations come to life.

Instructors also must wear a variety of hats when instructing. For example, the instructor needs to be a coach for students who are practicing skills and be an administrator when addressing program details. Being an effective instructor requires great versatility and an acute knowledge of what hat to wear and when to wear it!

CHAPTER 4, THEORIES AND CONCEPTS OF EDUCATION

Famous educational psychologists and their learning theories are reviewed. The philosophies from the 1800s through the 1900s have formed many of today's educational practices. Discussions regarding the "art versus the science of instruction" are deeply rooted in these philosophies. Key educational concepts, such as stimulus-response theory, are discussed within this chapter.

CHAPTER 5, BEHAVIORAL OBJECTIVES, LESSON PLANS, AND CURRICULUM

The introduction of Chapter 5 begins with an analogy. The analogy involves building a lesson plan as you would build a house. A house is built using a detailed set of blueprints (i.e., the lesson plan). The lesson presentation is centered on the behavioral objectives and the lesson plan. If the lesson plan is poorly constructed, chances are the lesson presentation will be poorly constructed.

Behavioral objectives are discussed extensively throughout this book. A lesson plan uses behavioral objectives to create the lesson presentation. The lesson's AV aids, teaching methods, handouts, facility setup, and examinations are identified in the lesson plan. Once a lesson plan is constructed, it becomes a component of the training institute's curriculum.

CHAPTER 6, MULTIMEDIA SYSTEMS AND EDUCATIONAL RESOURCES

Motivating students is essential. Educational resources supplement an instructor's presentation. Based on the lesson's objectives, a variety of AV equipment and educational materials are available to instructors. Commonly used educational resources are reviewed in this chapter.

PowerPoint and computer multimedia systems require instructors to understand how to design, use, and troubleshoot their presentations. There is more to a multimedia presentation than just following an online wizard's help instructions! CD-ROM examples will allow you to develop and use high-quality educational programs.

CHAPTER 7, FACILITY AND CLASSROOM SETUP

The type of atmosphere that surrounds students can affect their ability to learn information. A room that is noisy, is too hot/cold, is poorly lit, and has limited restroom facilities can affect a student's learning experience. Different classroom setups are reviewed, based on the type of presentation that is being taught.

CHAPTER 8, TEACHING STRATEGIES AND METHODS

There are many ways to instruct emergency service training programs. Teaching methods that are used are a reflection of an instructor's personality. At the conclusion of this chapter, you should be able to make informed decisions about what teaching methods will work for you and which ones will not likely fit you as an instructor.

CHAPTER 9, PSYCHOMOTOR DEVELOPMENT

Learning a skill requires mental and physical abilities. This chapter outlines how students use cognitive, affective, and psychomotor objectives to perform physical tasks. Students learn skills at different rates. Instructors need to know when to urge students on to the next learning level. Ultimate skill perfection is attained at the mastery level. The mastery level becomes a goal for both the students and the instructors to attain.

CHAPTER 10, EVALUATION TOOLS

Students and instructors who view practical and written examinations as "evil devices" have a very narrow view of the educational process. Examinations (i.e., evaluations) are tools to assist a student and instructor identify a student's level of learning. An evaluation should be a learning experience.

Various forms of written examinations are reviewed. Each of the examination formats relies upon well written behavioral objectives. Exam questions are referenced for specific objectives.

Practical evaluations are reviewed. Writing scenarios and creating realistic settings become key factors in designing practical examinations.

CHAPTER 11, PROGRAM EVALUATION

Instead of evaluating a student's performance, this chapter identifies ways to evaluate the entire course. The goal of a program evaluation is to indicate where a program is and where it needs to be.

How valid are the examinations? What quality assurance mechanisms are in place during a training program? Who reviews a class's performance after it concludes? These kinds of probing questions need to be asked. This is not a typical evaluation chapter. The review of the evaluation concepts is from a viewpoint rarely addressed in emergency service training programs.

CHAPTER 12, INTERNET AND COMPUTER-BASED INSTRUCTION

This chapter is dedicated to cutting-edge computer technologies. State-of-the-art technologies, like virtual reality, are transforming the way training programs are being taught. Online Internet classrooms, multimedia hardware, interactive software programs, CD-ROM simulations, and computer-based games are available to instructors.

Computers assist students and instructors explore resources and knowledge beyond the traditional classrooms. The Internet's history and future are reviewed. How to effectively use the Internet is discussed in detail.

CHAPTER 13, REALISM CONCEPTS

Adult learners need realism. The closer a lesson presentation comes to real-life situations the greater the learning experience is for the students.

Creating realism is more than just using cosmetic products to simulate an injury. It requires the right atmosphere, an appropriately written scenario, a patient actor who can act out the scenario, and the appropriate use of cosmetic-based products. Whether it is a two-story burn building or a simulated vehicle accident, realism concepts can create an enriched educational experience for students and instructors.

CHAPTER 14, LEGAL ASPECTS OF INSTRUCTION

For any emergency profession, instructors need to recognize the potential liabilities associated with a training program. Students who are permanently injured in a training program activity may sue both the instructor and the training institute. This chapter reviews the significant legal issues that instructors may encounter during a training program.

CHAPTER 15, PROGRAM ADMINISTRATION

The behind-the-scenes personnel often determine a training program's success or failure! How a program is planned, advertised, coordinated, and evaluated is the responsibility of the program administrator. How administration components are incorporated into a training program is discussed within this chapter.

Intended Uses of This Book

Whether you are a new instructor or a seasoned veteran, this textbook contains vital educational material designed for all emergency service instructors. Examples that are used are not from a home economics course; instead, they are from actual or simulated emergency situations.

Emergency services are dynamic. Whether it is EMS, fire, or rescue, new concepts and techniques are constantly being introduced. Instructors convey these innovative concepts in their training programs. How an instructor presents lesson material affects how students will learn life-saving concepts. This book provides instructors with the necessary instructional skills to make learning experiences interesting and motivational.

This book is intended to be a primary instructional reference for all emergency service instructors.

Summary

The last component in every chapter is the chapter's summary. The key concepts of the chapter are condensed into a few paragraphs.

The entire educational process is interrelated. This interrelationship is introduced in this chapter. However, the magnitude of the interrelationships cannot be appreciated until reading each of the chapters and seeing the actual interlinking relationships.

This book is a reference manual for instructors. Use it as a guide to enhance your lesson presentation. Ponder, discuss, investigate, and create innovative educational programs. Use this book as your guide to become the best instructor you can be. The greatest gift an instructor possesses is the ability to influence the many instead of the few.

Enjoy and read on so that you can become the best instructor that you can be!

Chapter 2
Adult Learners and Their Characteristics

➤ OBJECTIVES

- Define the term *andragogy*.
- Identify concepts associated with andragogy.
- Identify the term *pedagogy* and explain how it relates to andragogy.
- Identify the characteristics associated with an adult learner.
- Define the term *paradigm* and discuss how paradigms influence the learning process.
- Identify learning characteristics associated with all learners.
- Define, discuss, and explore the use of learning style inventory assessments.
- Explore and define the different types of students found in emergency service training programs.
- Define the dominant ego patterns displayed by adult learners.
- Identify motivational tendencies for emergency service personnel.
- Identify, define, and discuss literacy and reading comprehension abilities of adult learners.
- Define the ways of determining the mixture of the students in a training program.
- Identify the influence that noneducational factors play in training programs.
- Define methods for designing the training curriculum around the class mixture.

Today's EMS classes are composed of a unique melting pot of students. . . . it could be said that EMS training courses often meet and exceed the concepts of mainstreaming.

William D. McClincy, 1988[1]

Emergency service programs contain a melting pot of students. As an instructor, you should expect to find a variety of personality traits, learning characteristics, ages, educational backgrounds, and lifetime

---

[1]William McClincy, "Learning About the Learners," *Pennsylvania Department of Health Instructor Newsletter* (Harrisburg: The Department, 1988).

experiences for students in most emergency service classrooms. These factors create a unique mixture of students for an instructor to motivate.

The concept of mainstreaming, places slow learners and mentally/ physically challenged individuals into a classroom with nonchallenged students. What does this concept have to do with emergency service training programs? Educational institutions have a legal obligation to provide educational opportunities to these students (see Chapter 14, Americans with Disability Act). An instructor must be able to adapt and motivate students who have diminished or depressed learning skills, while motivating the other students.

The majority of students who attend emergency service training programs can be categorized as adult learners. Educational researchers have identified traits associated with adult learners. The term *andragogy* identifies characteristics associated with adult learning. Referred to as the Apostle of Andragogy, also known as the Father of Adult Education, Malcolm Knowles defined characteristics associated with an adult learner.[2] He discovered that adults have specific learning needs and motivations. Although the adult learner concepts have been critically reviewed and debated, Knowles's adult learning principles are widely found in today's educational programs.

This chapter looks at adult learning characteristics. Questions such as "Who are the learners?" and "How do students learn?" will be addressed. Additional aspects of adult learners will be identified and examined. The key for an instructor is to identify a learner's characteristics and build a lesson that will meet the needs of each student.

Andragogy and Pedagogy

In 1973 Malcolm Knowles published a book entitled *The Adult Learner: A Neglected Species.* This text described characteristics associated with adult learners and compared them to pedagogy characterists, which is learning associated with children. In his 1984 book *Andragogy in Action: Applying Modern Principles of Adult Education,* he amended his position regarding the differences between adult and child learning. Knowles identifies five assumptions for adult learners:

1. Adults tend to be self-directed and should be guided to discover information on their own.
2. Adults bring enriched experiences to the classroom. Activities that use these life experiences should be encouraged.
3. Adult learners have a readiness and are eager to learn.
4. Adult learners want to be able to apply the knowledge and skills into their daily work. They tend to be problem-centered learners, as opposed to adolescent learners who prefer structured, lecture-based presentations.
5. Adult learners have an interpersonal desire to better themselves.[3]

---

[2]Malcolm Knowles: Apostle of Andragogy, nlu.nl.edu/ace/Resources/Knowles.html. This discussion is taken from Malcolm Knowles, *The Adult Learner: A Neglected Species,* rev. ed. (Houston, Tex.: Gulf, 1990).

[3]Malcolm Knowles, et al., *Andragogy in Action: Applying Modern Principles of Adult Education* (San Francisco: Jossey Bass, 1984).

These principles are not unique to adult learners, as critics of Knowles are quick to point out. Many of the characteristics of adult learners can and should be identified with adolescent learners. Simply, there are not significant differences in the learning styles between adult and adolescent learners, as was once believed. Knowles states that both groups should be viewed separately. He notes that adult learners prefer experiential learning situations, while adolescent learners tend to depend upon an instructor to tell them how to learn. These adult education principles have impacted today's management of adult education courses. Instructors should gain an understanding of these perspectives that motivate adult learners and incorporate them into their lesson presentations.

FORCED LEARNING

If there is one fact that an instructor must be aware of, it is this: *"adult learners cannot be forced to learn."* Many adult learners are forced into training programs against their will or best judgement. These "forced" students do not follow Knowles's adult learning principles. Adult learners who are forced to attend a training program usually display a poor attitude and lack motivation in their classroom activities. As discussed later in this chapter, instructors need to get to know who their students are. Knowing that students are mandated to attend a training program should cause changes in an instructor's lesson plan. For example, an instructor should not expect to be overly successful with a discussion format in a classroom of unmotivated individuals.

Adult learners who are placed in a forced learning situation tend to have a poor learning experience. To make a meaningful learning experience for this type of student, the instructor must redirect the student's motivation for attending the program. Dealing with adult learners in a critical learning situation is explored in "Ego States: Transactional Analysis," a section later in this chapter.

LEARNING BY DOING

A basic educational concept associated with adult learners and adolescent learners is the concept of learning by doing. In Chapter 4 of this book, the Father of Education, John Dewey, outlines his pragmatic educational philosophy. Pragmatists believe that learning by doing is the principal basis of learning, regardless of the subject. Years of research show that students learn and retain information best when they become active participants in the learning process; students learn by doing! When students use knowledge in actual settings, the learning and retention of knowledge and/or skills approach the highest level of attainment. The concept of learning by doing is illustrated by Figure 2-1.

Identified in the chart, the closer a lesson comes to the "real thing," the higher is the degree of learning and retention of the information. The concept of learning by doing forms a key educational foundation. Acknowledging the significance of this fact, instructors should build their lesson

Relationships of Learning

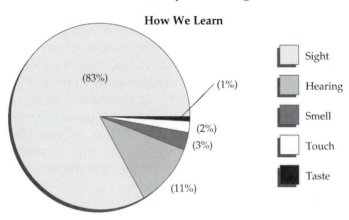

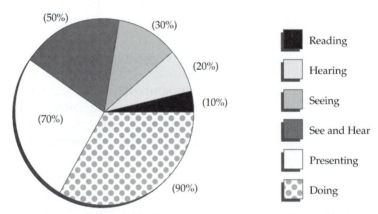

Figure 2-1
The top chart shows
how students learn
and the bottom
chart shows the
retention of the
information.

*Source: Adapted from materials found in the Pennsylvania Department of
Health Rescue Instructor Curriculum (Harrisburg: The Department, 1983).*

plans around this concept. Even with a well-developed lesson plan, not
every presentation will attain high levels of learning and retention. A student's motivation, the type of lesson material, and the overall curriculum
design can limit the level of learning and retention. Instructors should
strive to make their lessons as close to the real thing as possible. This requires time, patience, and motivation on an instructor's part. If students are
going to attain a positive learning experience, the instructor needs to design
a lesson presentation that pushes toward the higher levels of learning.

ADULT LEARNERS AND REALISM

Adult learners need to have realistic, practical, and knowledgeable lessons.
Adult learners can have difficulty imagining a piece of equipment, responding to a written scenario, or attempting to perform a skill within a
pretend scenario. Figure 2-1 shows that when adults are given a situation
to which they can practically apply their knowledge, high levels of learn-

ing and retention occur. Thus, the closer an instructor can make a situation to real life, the better the learning experience will be for the students.

In Chapter 13, realistic concepts are discussed at length. Numerous realistic techniques can be used to enhance a learning experience. Realistic techniques allow adult learners to become more involved in contrived situations, which increases their learning potential.

When introducing a new piece of equipment or a skill, an instructor must show the equipment or demonstrate the skill before fully presenting the topic. Educationally, this is known as making referent contact, which will be discussed in Chapters 8 and 9. This initial demonstration is designed to visually show the information to the students. Students will model their behaviors from this initial visual image.

To maximize the learning experience, adding realism to a lesson can improve both learning and retention. Instead of pretending, the students experience "almost real" life situations in the classroom.

Adult Learners and Grades

Bear in mind Knowles's fifth andragogy principle, "Adult learners have an interpersonal desire to better themselves." Generally, adult learners are attending a training program to better their knowledge of a particular subject. The majority of adult learners are not in competition to attain the highest score on an examination. Adult learners' main motivation is to learn the information so they can use the information in their daily lives. This is not to say that there will not be students who are competitive and will want to get the best score in class. They're out there!

An instructor should establish a minimum level of expected performance for his adult learners. However, too often, instructors and students get caught up in the attainment of scores on examinations. Adult learners who are motivated to learn because they desire knowledge tend to do well throughout their course, including their exams. Students whose sole motivation is something other than the improvement of their knowledge (i.e., job promotion, social status) often experience difficulty throughout their learning experience. Students' internal motivations are an essential element in not only their learning but throughout their life experiences. In the next section, an individual's internal motivation is further identified.

GNS and Adult Learners

Behavioral researchers Hackman and Oldham developed an assessment tool called the JDS (Job Diagnostic Survey).[4] JDS measures the degree of match between individuals and their jobs. The assessment breaks job assignments into critical and psychological components. The JDS assessment uses a moderator known as GNS. *GNS* stands for growth need strength. GNS measures the psychological needs of an individual. It assesses the

---

[4]R. J. Hackman and G. R. Oldham, *Work Redesign* (Reading, Mass.: Addison-Wesley, 1980).

strong need for personal challenge, growth, accomplishment, learning, and attainment of professional development.

GNS measures the degree of an individual's internal motivation. Individuals with high internal motivation will find a job assignment or task challenging. Individuals with diminished growth needs tend to be less aggressive to pursue growth opportunities. Low GNS individuals are content with the status quo and will be reluctant to accept change.

What impact does GNS have on educational programs? Students who exhibit high GNS will be bored by activities that do not challenge them. Conversely, students with diminished GNS will feel overwhelmed by activities that challenge their abilities. Low GNS students are content with knowing the basics and will have a diminished classroom motivation. Low GNS students will not seek out learning opportunities and are not likely to be active participants in independent discovery activities.

Instructors whose students exhibit diminished GNS should use presentations that are informative and motivating but do not overly challenge a student's abilities. Students with diminished GNS should be partnered with individuals who exhibit high GNS. Structured course activities and classroom discussions would be helpful to open a dialogue between high and diminished GNS students.

Data collected in independent assessments of EMS personnel indicate that emergency personnel are prone to exhibit low GNS characteristics.[5] Instructors should listen to their students' dialogue during classroom interactions. Students with high GNS will desire additional information, while diminished GNS students will express feelings of being overwhelmed and overly challenged by the course materials.

A conscious awareness of an individual's GNS orientation is necessary to improve the GNS score. Then planning and practicing activities that challenge the individual's abilities, over time, can enhance the GNS score.

Paradigm

In his book, *The Structure of Scientific Revolution*, Thomas Kuhn defined the obscure term *paradigm*. He redefined the term as it related to behaviors that he observed in scientists while they worked on scientific investigations. He defines a paradigm as "a constellation of concepts, values, perceptions and practices shared by a community which forms a particular vision of reality that is the basis of the way a community organizes itself."[6]

Kuhn discovered that scientists often did not accept information that did not fit their perception of how it should fit. He found that paradigms acted as a filter of incoming information. In order for scientists to "see" new information, they had to be willing to change their perception of what the finding should be. These filtering effects of paradigms can be seen among

---

[5]W. D. McClincy, "Turnover Intentions of Emergency Personnel" (master's thesis, Gannon University, Erie, 1994).

[6]Kuhn, Thomas S., *The Structure of Scientific Revolutions*, Second Edition, Enlarged, (Chicago: The University of Chicago Press, 1970).

our daily lives. At home, work, or in education programs there is a set of rules of performance.

Paradigms have a significant influence on the educational process. Educators create behavioral objectives to predict changes in a student's behavior. When an instructor encounters a student's behavior that is not expected, the instructor can explore the behavior or dismiss it because it does not fit the established curricula. New ideas and perspectives are often ignored because they are not contained in the lesson plan. Instructors should plan activities that encourage students to explore and seek out new paradigms.

Ego States: Transactional Analysis

How adults learn and react to information is often dependent upon their state of mind or Ego State. Eric Berne is the founder of transactional analysis (TA).[7] TA is a form of social psychology that focuses on external and internal psychological states. There are three ego states:

1. Parent
2. Child
3. Adult

At any point during a class, an adult learner or instructor can display any of these characteristics. Transactional analysts note that adults are really three people inside the body of one person. Each ego state has positive and negative aspects. An instructor should listen to a student's comments and try to identify the ego state from which the student is responding.

The child ego state deals with emotions. In this state, one can be playful, loving, creative, caring, fearful, angry, sad, disruptive, and so forth. Students or instructors may be 35 or 40 years old but act and react to situations as if they were 5 or 6 years old. Depending on the classroom activity, acting in a child ego state can be beneficial. For example, while participating in an interactive classroom game, a child ego state can bring excitement to the activity. Unfortunately the child ego state causes adults to react inappropriately to some situations. Thus, many adults hide their child ego state and favor their parent or adult ego states.

Often characterized as the tape recorder ego state, the parent ego state tends to be overly critical and rigid and is based on prejudged values. In the parent ego state, there is a defined boundary. Cross a line, consequences will result. The parent ego state constantly "plays" prerecorded attitudes and opinions. These tapes are based on their parents' and their parents' parents' attitudes and values. For example, an instructor in a critical parent ego state might tell students how activities shall be conducted regardless of their input; tell them what is correct or incorrect, "I'm right and you're

---

[7]Claude Steiner, Ph.D., www.claudesteiner.com/ta.htm; Gram Barnes, ed., *Transactional Analysis after Eric Barnes: Teaching and Practices of Three TA Studies* (New York: Harper's College Press, 1977); Interview with family therapist David Glenn, M.A. Ed., Meadville, Pa., September 2000.

wrong"; and even attempt to belittle students, or vice versa students to the instructor, in front of the class. These examples show a subparent ego state known as the critical parent (also known as the pig parent). There also is a nurturing parent ego state, which is supportive and protective. It is the nurturing parent ego state that provides positive "strokes." TA defines strokes as physical touching or verbal rewards. Strokes can be either positive or negative, but regardless of the type of strokes, Berne notes that individuals need strokes to survive. Individuals who do not receive positive strokes will seek negative strokes, just to be recognized. Instructors should try to provide students with positive rewards whenever it is possible.

The third ego state is the adult ego state. This ego state responds to situations in a logical and rational manner and tends to be a nonemotional state. This state has been likened to a computer! Facts and information are used to make logical decisions. Making decisions from a logical perspective is not always advantageous. The adult ego state is responsible for the control of the parent and child ego states. Changing interactions from a parent or child ego state is possible by using the adult ego state.

Instructors will encounter a variety of ego states in their classes. How instructors communicate information to their students is frequently determined by how they respond to a student's question or verbal statement. TA defines successful communication as a "complementary transaction" (see Exhibit 2-1). Transactions flow from the three ego states. For example, if instructors respond from a parent ego state, they expect a child ego state response. If the response instead comes from an adult ego state, the transaction becomes "crossed" and results in ineffective communication. Continual crossed transactions can lead to hostile situations occurring and a total breakdown in all communication (see Exhibit 2-2).

The use of TA can be seen in handling day-to-day conversations in the workplace and in daily life activities. Instructors must be able to listen, understand, and then respond to students by using complementary transactions and avoiding crossing transactions. Keeping an open line of communication between students and instructors ensures effective information exchange within a training program.

Learning Styles

Adults or adolescent learners will favor a particular way to learn. Some may prefer reading from textbooks and completing homework assignments, while others prefer less textbook work and more hands-on activities. These differences are actually a reflection of an individual's learning style.

The National Standard U.S. Department of Transportation 1994 EMT-B Curriculum identifies three learning characteristics: auditory, visual, and kinesthetic (AVK).[8] A fourth learning characteristic, tactile, is incorporated into the kinesthetic characteristic, although it is actually considered to be a

---

[8]U.S. Department of Transportation 1994 National Standard Curriculum EMT-B (Washington, D.C.: U.S. Government Printing Office, 1994).

Exhibit 2-1

Examples of Transactions

1. Adult (teacher) to Adult (student)

Teacher: During the last class I asked everyone to try to complete the homework assignment. Did anyone have any difficulty on the first section?

James: I do not completely understand the friction loss between the two types of hose that were described in the first section.

2. Adult (teacher) to Parent Ego (student)

Teacher: During the last class I asked everyone to try to complete the homework assignment. Did anyone have any difficulty on the first section?

Ted: I do not understand why we have to learn these friction loss ratios when we are going to be interior firefighters.

3. Parent (teacher) to Adult (student)

Teacher: Jeff, I told you the answer to that question last week. Weren't you paying attention again?

Jeff: I was confused by the homework material and I didn't seem to arrive at the same answer.

4. Adult (teacher) to Child (student)

Teacher: John, what answer did you get for the friction loss question in Section 1?

John: I didn't answer the question because the information wasn't covered in the book and I didn't understand your notes.

separate characteristic. These AVK learning characteristics influence how a student learns and retains information.

Auditory (A) learners "hear" the information, visual (V) learners "see" the information, kinesthetic (K) learners learn through physical movements, and tactile learners learn by touch. Students tend to favor one or two of these learning methods. How do these learning characteristics affect how students learn and retain information? Let's look at each characteristic.

Visual learners want to see the instructor teach. They will watch the instructor's movements in the classroom. Visual learners will mimic their skill performance after the instructor's demonstration. They need to see the key points highlighted on a dry image board or overhead transparency.

Exhibit 2-2

Crossed Responses

Adult (teacher) responding to a Parent (student) response

Teacher: Your rescue squad has responded to the scene
            of an MVA, car into a tree. One person is trapped
            inside on the driver's side. Due to the damage,
            none of the doors open and the passenger side is
            pushed against some trees. How would you gain
            access to the person? State the tools that you
            would use if the power hydraulic tool were
            broken.

Mitch: This is a dumb scenario. I have never had the tool
            not work. So I would use the power hydraulic tool
            in any case.

Teacher: Yes, this is a scenario that a rescuer tries to avoid
            by good preventative maintenance. However, the
            question asks for tools of access. The power hy-
            draulic tool takes time to set up. By definition,
            access is to be a quick entry into the vehicle to be
            able to access the patient and to determine the
            degree of entrapment. The power hydraulic tool
            is "broken" because it is not the tool of choice for
            this scenario.

Multimedia presentations, videotapes, and charts/diagrams are preferred by a visual learner. Interestingly, visual learners do not prefer learning material from textbooks.

It is actually the auditory learner who prefers textbook learning.[9] But "hearing" the information should not be associated only with an instructor's presentation. Auditory learners silently sound out words as they read from a textbook. Listening to themselves reading helps them retain the book's information. Auditory learners are good listeners and pick up information by watching and listening to discussions. The auditory learner prefers hearing presentations that involve the instructor and students in audible classroom discussions.

The kinesthetic or tactile learner prefers learning situations that require their physical participation. Kinesthetic learners want to "do." They do not want to listen to a lecture or participate in a complex textbook activity.

---

[9]Marcia Conner, *Wave Technologies*, "Learning: The Critical Technology." Learning Styles and Assessments, www.learnactivity.com/body_styles.html. 1995/1999.

Luckily, most emergency service training programs include a lot of hands-on training, which favors the kinesthetic/tactile learner.

Instructors should try to incorporate each AVK characteristic into their classroom presentations. This will help students learn the material by using their preferred learning style.

In addition to the AVK learning styles, other specialized learning-style inventories can help students and instructors identify their individual learning behaviors.

Dr. Richard M. Felder and Barbara A. Soloman from North Carolina State University have developed a written assessment called the Index of Learning Styles (ILS).[10] The ILS measures four learning traits: active/reflective, sensing/intuitive, visual/verbal, and sequential/global. Active learners tend to retain and understand the information by doing something with it. In contrast, reflective learners prefer to quietly think about the information. Similar comparisons are made between the other assessment components. A version of the assessment can be taken via the Internet at www2.ncsu.edu/unity/lockers/users/f/felder/public/ILSdir/ilsweb.html

David Kolb has pioneered the use of the learning style inventory (LSI).[11] The LSI identifies four specific learning modes: concrete experience (learning from experiences and being sensitive to the feelings of others), reflective observation (observing and examining an issue from different perspectives), abstract conceptualization (analysis of issues, systemic planning, and developing an understanding of the information), and active experimentation (learning by doing, ability to get things done, and being a risk taker). Learners will pass through these phases as they learn information. Learners tend to develop preferences between the learning modes. The LSI groups the learning modes into learning styles. The LSI types are accommodating, assimilating, converging, and diverging. Figure 2-2 shows the learning modes and learning styles.

A learner with an assimilating learning style prefers taking time to think about the information and learns best by reading, listening, and observing. The accommodating learner prefers learning by doing. "Just let me do it" is a commonly heard phrase. Accommodating learners prefer experiential learning situations and dislike sitting in lectures and doing book work. Converging learners prefer situations in which they can plan and use information to solve problems. A converging learner likes to be mentally challenged by the learning experience. The last learning style type is the diverging learner. Diverging learners look at information from a variety of viewpoints. They prefer brainstorming activities and watching the actions of other students.

An online version of the LSI assessment can be taken at: trgmcber.haygroup.com/learning/lsius.htm. There is a charge for this assessment.

---

[10]Richard M. Felder and Barbara A. Soloman, Learning Styles, Index of Learning Styles, www2.ncsu.edu/unity/lockers/users/f/felder/public/Learning_Styles.html, North Carolina State University, November 2000.

[11]David A. Kolb, *Experiential Learning: Experience as the Source of Learning and Development* (Upper Saddle River, N.J.: Prentice Hall, 1984); and David A. Kolb, *Learning Style Inventories*, 3rd ed. (Boston: Hay Resources Direct, 1999).

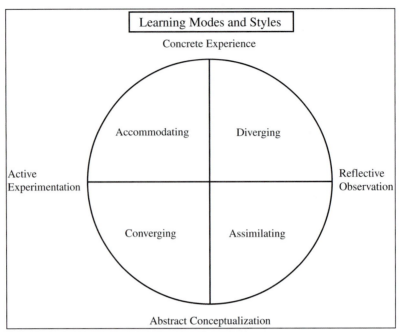

Figure 2-2
Learning modes and styles.

Source: Adapted from David Kolb's Learning Style Inventory, Version 3. © 1999, Hay Resources Direct.

Another popular assessment is the Myers-Briggs Type Indicator (MBTI).[12] This assessment is actually a personality profile assessment of a learner's affective domain. The four traits (called poles) assessed are extroversion (E)/introversion (I), sensing (S)/intuition (N), thinking (T)/feeling (F), and judging (J)/perception (P). A letter score is derived from the four traits. There are 16 possible scoring combinations (i.e., INFP or ESTJ). As an instructor, you might find it beneficial to identify your personality profile. An instructor's individual traits can affect how students learn information.

Identifying learning style types and personality characteristics can help students and instructors become effective learners and problem solvers. When conflicts of opinion occur in classrooms or in real-life situations they are often the result of different learning styles or personalities colliding. An instructor may prefer to use one learning style or personality trait while students prefer another style or trait. It is important to note these differences. Ideally, instructors should plan their lessons around the students' learning styles. But if conflicts of opinion occur, planned or unplanned, they can be opportunities to explore differing points of view, and as a result new information or applications are often identified.

Who Are the Students?

Students attending emergency service training programs are quite diversified. Age, gender, education, social background, economic status, career advancement, plus other factors influence students attending a training

---

[12] Isabel Briggs-Myers and Mary H. McCaulley, *Manual: A Guide to the Development and Use of the Myers-Briggs Type Indicator*, (Palo Alto, Calif.: Consulting Psychologists Press, 1985).

program. Let us look at these factors and how they influence emergency service training programs.

FORMAL EDUCATION BACKGROUND

For some students attending an emergency service training program, it may be their first formal training program since they graduated from high school. For other students it may have been only two or three years since their last training program. Then there are students enrolled who have never finished high school, and sitting next to them are students who are in college or are taking the training as part of their full-time employment. Quite a diversified group of students!

For the students who have been out of the training process for several years, reading and understanding textbook material, taking notes, and studying for tests can be overwhelming. Retraining, and often initial training, of good study and reading habits is as important as the lesson material.

Determining the students' educational background can help an instructor design lesson presentations around their needs. Instead of "talking over the heads" of the students, instructors can target their lesson presentations to the students' level of understanding.

SPECIALTY EDUCATION BACKGROUND

Students can bring a wealth of personal experience to emergency service training programs. An instructor should plan lesson activities around the experiences of the students.

Prerequisites to many training courses require previous training and certification. Unless an instructor asks students to verify their training, significant academic and safety circumstances can occur. For example, an advanced self-contained breathing apparatus (SCBA) course is being conducted. A prerequisite into the program is to have already completed a basic SCBA course. Two of the students have no formal SCBA training. When verbally asked by the instructor at the beginning of the class, the students did not disclose their lack of training. Only when the two are in the middle of the smokehouse does the instructor become aware that neither has any training.

Instructors need to do more than just ask their students. Validation of training credentials must be reviewed prior to a training program. The example also shows another trait commonly seen among adult learners; that trait is the influence of social pressure placed upon students by their peers.

SOCIAL BACKGROUND

Using the previous SCBA example, once the students are safely removed from the smokehouse environment, the instructor has a frank conversation with them. The instructor determines that the two students lied because of their "pride." Other members of their department had completed this advanced training and they were going to get the training at any cost. Societal pressure caused these two students to endanger themselves, the instructors, and the other students.

Often an instructor may know some of the students enrolled in their course. For instructors who teach high-risk courses (e.g., trench rescue, high-angle rescue, fire/rescue), it is critical to determine the social background of the students. Instructors should silently ask themselves, "From what societal background are the students that are attending the course?" Students driven by social pressures need to be counseled before they endanger themselves and other students. The middle of a high-risk practice session is not the time to identify these societally-driven students!

PHYSICAL CAPABILITIES

The opening paragraph of this chapter mentioned the concept of mainstreaming. The original intent of mainstreaming was to allow the physically challenged students access to elementary and secondary classrooms. What does mainstreaming have to do with emergency service training programs? The answer is, "a lot!"

In nearly every emergency service classroom, there are individuals with physical disabilities. Included are individuals with underlying medical conditions such as asthma, hypertension, cardiovascular abnormalities, diabetic conditions, recent major surgery, chronic back injuries, musculoskeletal injuries, vision or hearing impairment, and the list goes on. Many states require students to read and sign a functional job description statement. As discussed in Chapter 14, "Legal Aspects of Instruction," the functional job description details tasks and activities that will be expected from a student during a training program. When it is appropriate, reasonable accommodations must be afforded to the student.

Many physically handicapped students can perform skills if given a chance to modify the skill to meet their disability. Instructors should assist these students in their attempt to learn a skill. However, if the program is one that leads to state certification, most certification examinations cannot be extensively modified. States have an obligation to uphold the public trust that certified personnel are competent to perform the essential skills required by a specific task. All students must be made aware of the functional job description in the initial phases of a course.

Aside from physically handicapped students, there are additional handicaps that prevent students from learning. The most significant one is a broad category titled learning disabilities.

LEARNING DISABLED STUDENTS

The term *learning disabled* carries many definitions. These include dyslexia, illiteracy, slow learners, and other reading disabilities. Many adults do not know why they cannot learn; they have always had difficulty learning and have accepted their learning disability.

National literacy statistics reveal that an estimated 10 to 20 percent of the U.S. population over the age of 20 is considered functionally illiterate.[13] Many of these adults learn to cope with their illiteracy. Not even their family members, friends, or employers can tell that the individual has a reading disability.

Depending on how much formal education adult learners have, they may not have ever had a diagnosis of a learning disability. Their grade school or high school teachers may have told them "they weren't trying or working hard enough." Many teachers had large classes and could not spend the time to find out why the student was not learning. Other teachers were not trained to recognize a learning disability, much less to help the student overcome the disability. Years later, emergency service instructors are presented with these same students who are not dumb but have an undiagnosed learning disability. The million-dollar question: "What does the emergency service instructor do with a learning disabled student?"

Coping with the Learning Disabled Student

Most emergency service instructors do not have degrees in educational psychology or in special education. How can instructors deal with students who have a learning disability? The first step is to make sure that the students realize they have a learning disability. If they do not acknowledge that they have a problem, there is little that an instructor can do to assist them. However, if they are aware they have problems reading or comprehending material, then a local reading specialist (e.g., high school, vocational school, community outreach reading program) should be contacted and a formal diagnosis made. Depending on the diagnosis, students often can seek remedial training to cope with their disabilities. Unless professionally trained, an emergency service instructor should rely on the community's educational resources to assist students to improve their learning skills.

Often, some learning disabilities, such as dyslexia, cannot be easily corrected. Only through professionally supervised training does an individual learn to cope with such a disability.

Dyslexia One of the most widely known learning disabilities is dyslexia. A student with dyslexia incorrectly interprets the information due to a variety of physiological or neurological causes. An extreme example of a dyslexic learner, with a sight information abnormality, can be seen in the following passage:

> *Normal: The emergency vehicles should be placed a minimum of 100'*
> *away from the scene of a vehicle that is on fire.*
> *Dyslexic: hte emergncey hiclvees houlds eb placde a miminum of 001'*
> *away mrof hte csene fo a vehcile htat is on fire.*

---

[13]Second estimate. National Institute of Education, U.S. Department of Education (Washington, D.C.: Office of Vocational and Adult Education, June 1990).

Every dyslexic's diagnosis is different. Not every word is misunderstood. An individual's dyslexia can be related to sight, hearing, psychomotor coordination, and other inputs or outputs.

Educational specialists train students with dyslexia to unscramble the words or symbols so that they make sense. The critical factor is time. It takes twice the time for a dyslexic individual to read or hear a passage and then unscramble the meaning of the passage. Thus, if a student has dyslexia, the student should be permitted extra time on examinations to unscramble the information.

Slow Learner/Poor Reader A student who falls into this category presents a different challenge for emergency service instructors. An instructor can provide assistance to these students, while still teaching the rest of the class. To do this, the instructor can modify the lesson plan, worksheets, and even the textbook for the slow learner or poor reader.

This does not require lengthy modifications to the lesson material. First, the instructor must identify any students who have a problem reading or understanding the material. This is accomplished by several different approaches. Many times, students will initiate a conversation with their instructors to discuss their inability to understand the material. Or the instructor will openly announce during a class session that any student who is having a problem understanding the material should see the instructor privately after the class session ends. Or the instructor can call for a private counseling session with a student who has performed poorly on a unit examination. Before modifying the lesson material, the student must realize that a problem exists. Then the instructor can react appropriately to the student's learning difficulties.

The next step is to provide the necessary assistance to the student. There are several approaches that an instructor can use to modify the course materials. The instructor's reaction must be proportional to the student's disability. If the student cannot understand the textbook material, the instructor should try to identify a textbook that has a lower reading level. If the student's problem stems from too many distractions during an examination—for example, peer pressure or time constraints—offer the student the option of taking the test alone in a quiet room and extend the time for the examination. Identifying a workbook and assigning problems can be beneficial to the student. Extra practice sessions can be offered for those students having a problem developing their skill proficiency. For instructors who have appropriate training, conducting remedial one-to-one training sessions with individual students may be another alternative. If several students in a course are having the same difficulty, the instructor may want to consider modifying the lesson plan to include group activities. These students can be paired together, so they can jointly learn the material.

Any of the previous approaches can be used. The instructor must be able to design the modification to meet the student's needs. Not every student requires one-to-one teaching. Instructors will identify students in their programs with these learning disabilities. Given the right assistance, an instructor will see these students performing as well as the other students in the course. Seeing these students performing well will make any extra instructional time and effort worthwhile.

AGE

An emergency service instructor can expect student ages to range from 16 to 76. With this wide age diversity, an instructor must become sensitive to the needs of the different students.

Younger Students

Often these students still think they are in high school. They challenge the instructor, not for the knowledge benefit, but for the disruption benefit. Instructors spend more time dealing with these disruptive students instead of being able to teach the class. On the other hand, many younger students are highly motivated, excited to have a new training experience, actively participate in classroom activities, and become model students. An instructor should expect either reaction from a group of younger students and be prepared to control the classroom.

Older Students

In contrast to younger students, older students have their own unique challenges. Older students bring their vast knowledge and experience to the classroom. An instructor can tap this information and use it to the class's benefit. However, older students often relate the information in a "war story" format, which can be distracting. Additionally, they can use this knowledge to challenge the instructor. The phrases "I remember when . . . ," "I don't recall ever needing to use that procedure . . . ," or "I've never had that situation in all my years . . ." are challenges to an instructor. Whatever the response, the instructor often will not be judged by the answer but by the style used to answer the question.

Instructors should respond in a sincere, nonthreatening manner and with a nonbelittling demeanor to all students, not just the older students. Instructors may find that the older students do not like the word *new* and may not be excited with improved techniques (in other words, change) or will not be the best students for group activities. These are challenges that should be expected when teaching an emergency service program.

EXPERIENCE

Identified with the older adult students, these students bring a variety of experiences to the classroom. In contrast, the younger students have little or no firsthand experience. The students caught in the middle fit both ends of the spectrum; some have a wealth of experience while others have little.

Experience ends up being another determinant in the construction of the lesson plan. Students who have countless firsthand experiences require less basic information than do students who have little or no knowledge or experience. Knowing that the class comprises a mixture of students helps an instructor to balance the lesson plan for all.

To balance a lesson plan is to provide information to all the students, not just to one group of students. Too much basic material will bore the seasoned students but will be motivating for the new students. Conversely, directing the lesson to the seasoned students will provide little information to the new students. Some instructors have found it useful in a mixed class to design group activities to pair new students with seasoned students. Through the instructor's careful coordination and foresight, the learning experience can become a positive learning experience for both groups. Determining the experience level of the students is a key piece in designing the lesson plan.

The previous sections have looked at types of student characteristics found in emergency service training programs. An instructor identifies the types of students enrolled in a course in order to design the lesson material. The process of defining the students is known as determining the class mix.

The Class Mix

The components of the class mix have already been identified. The "who" question answered many of the class mix questions. The students come from varied educational levels and social backgrounds and may have physical or learning disabilities, major age differences, and different levels of experience. But *why* are they attending the program? The "why" answer may be the most significant response to any question that is asked.

Already identified in the andragogy section of this chapter, motivation is the primary learning component for an adult learner. Motivation is also the primary "why" question. "Why are you taking this course?" Most adult learners who are forced to learn information perform poorly. Knowing that students are being mandated to attend the training program allows an instructor to design the lesson plan for that group of students.

Another part of the "why" question should evaluate the expectations of the students. Some students do not know what to expect from a training program, while other students have high expectations. An instructor should design a program that will meet the expectations of the students.

Asking the "who" and "why" questions before a program starts can define the class mix. This information allows the instructor to design the lesson plan for a specific group of students. The next section looks at how the class mix questions can be asked through the use of a preenrollment form.

Assembling the Class Mix

Determining the class mix before a program begins helps an instructor make the lessons for a specific group of students. To find out who is in the class, a preenrollment questionnaire can be a useful evaluation tool.

The preenrollment questionnaires (Exhibits 2-3 and 2-4) use the "who" and "why" questions to formulate the questionnaire. Since EMS- and fire/

Exhibit 2-3

EMS Program Questionnaire

DIRECTIONS: This questionnaire is designed to assist your instructors in preparing lesson materials. You are asked to complete the survey questions and return the form in the enclosed envelope. Your answers will help design the lessons that will be used in your class.

NAME:_____

ADDRESS: _____

_____

PHONE NUMBER: _____

1. Circle your highest level of education:

   Fewer than 10, 11, 12, 13, 14, 15, 16; over 16

2. Circle the years of experience in EMS:

   Less than 1, 2, 3, 4, 5, 6, 7, 8, 9, 10; over 10

3. ____ Yes ____ No I am a member of an ambulance service.

   (If Yes, name the service) _____

4. ____ Yes ____ No Do you have any physical or reading difficulties that would require special assistance? (If yes, please explain.)

   _____

   _____

   _____

   _____

rescue-based programs have specific knowledge and experience requirements, the two examples that are illustrated reflect these requirements.

Incorporated into the questionnaires is an element of confidentiality. The purpose of the class mix questionnaire is to determine the mix of students enrolled in a training program. Often these questionnaires are used as screening mechanisms for training programs. These screening questionnaires push the limits of the federal antidiscrimination law and other associated federal laws. The questionnaire is designed to provide class mix information. Any other use is against its intended purpose.

Exhibit 2-3 (cont'd.)

EMS Program Questionnaire

5. From the following list identify the previous EMS training programs that you have attended.

___ Basic CPR	___ Emerg. Responder	___ First Responder (State Certified)
___ EMT Basic	___ EMT Defib	___ EMT Intermediate
___ Paramedic I	___ Paramedic II	___ Paramedic
___ PHTLS	___ BTLS	___ PALS
___ ACLS	___ Dispatcher	___ Vehicle Rescue
___ Haz Mat R&I	___ CISD	___ Other
___ Other _____	___ Other _____	___ Other _____

6. Please explain briefly why you are enrolled in this training program:

   _____

   _____

7. What do you expect to learn from this course? _____

   _____

8. How did you hear about the course? _____

   _____

   _____

Please mail or return this form to the primary instructor or course coordinator as soon as possible. Your input will help form the lesson plans for the program.

THANK YOU for your help.

Summary

This chapter has examined the features associated with adult learners. College courses, textbooks, and research projects are devoted to exploring and developing an understanding of the adult learners. Key principles associated with adult learners have been identified and explained in detail.

Adult learners bring a variety of learning experiences and emotional states to a classroom. Each experience, or emotional state, presents a different challenge to an instructor. Instructors determine the perspective that the student is coming from and respond appropriately to the student's actions.

Exhibit 2-4

Fire/Rescue Questionnaire

DIRECTIONS: This questionnaire is designed to assist your instructors in preparing lesson materials. You are asked to complete the survey questions and return the form in the enclosed envelope. Your answers will help design the lessons that will be used in your class.

NAME:_____

ADDRESS: _____

_____

PHONE NUMBER: _____

1. Circle your highest level of education:

   Less than 10, 11, 12, 13, 14, 15, 16; over 16

2. Circle the years of experience in EMS:

   Less than 1, 2, 3, 4, 5, 6, 7, 8, 9, 10; over 10

3. ____ Yes ____ No   I am a member of an ambulance service.

   (If Yes, name the service) _____

4. ____ Yes ____ No   Do you have any physical or reading difficulties that would require special assistance? (If Yes, please explain.)

   _____

   _____

   _____

   _____

Some students enrolled in emergency service programs have physical or mental disabilities that hinder their learning experience. Instructors work with these students and integrate them into the main class activities, a technique called mainstreaming. In some cases, modifying the lesson materials to allow an improved understanding of the material is required.

To learn what type of students are enrolled in a program, an instructor determines the class mix. Using the adult learning principles and adult characteristics, an opinion questionnaire identifies the mix of the students in a class. This allows the instructor to design the lesson to meet the needs of the students.

Exhibit 2-4 (cont'd.)

Fire/Rescue Questionnaire

5. From the following list identify the previous EMS training programs that you have attended.

___ Basic CPR	___ AFA	___ First Responder (State Certified)
___ EMT Basic	___ FFI cert	___ Fundamentals of Firefighting
___ Basic Firefighter	___ FF II cert	___ Structures I or II
___ Hydraulic	___ Haz Mat Respd	___ SCBA Basic or Advanced
___ ICS Orientation	___ Dispatcher	___ Vehicle Rescue
___ Haz Mat R&I	___ CISD	___ High Angle Rescue
___ Other _____	___ Other _____	___ Confined Space/Trench Rescue

6. Please explain briefly why you are enrolled in this training program:

_____

_____

7. What do you expect to learn from this course? _____

_____

8. How did you hear about the course? _____

_____

_____

Please mail or return this form to the primary instructor or course coordinator as soon as possible. Your input will help form the lesson plans for the program.

THANK YOU for your help.

Teaching adult learners is challenging and rewarding. Because of the adult student's self-motivation and willingness to learn information, teaching adult education courses is enjoyable for both the students and for the instructor. Working with people whose sole desire is to better themselves makes teaching worthwhile.

Chapter 3

Instructors and Their Characteristics

➤ **OBJECTIVES**

- Define *instruction.*
- Define *instructor.*
- Define an instructor's qualities.
- Identify roles assumed by an instructor.
- Identify characteristics associated with successful instructors.
- Compare positive instructional characteristics with those that are considered poor or ineffective.
- Identify the mental roles that an instructor plays during the delivery of material to the students.
- Define basic principles of instruction.
- Summarize organizational approaches that can be used to improve an instructor's presentation.

Instructional Motto

A s an instructor I will:

- Be who I am and know my limitations.
- Possess the knowledge and skill necessary for credibility.
- Respect the students' knowledge, experience, and abilities.
- Understand the learning style differences among students.
- Practice and use the learning formula in my presentations.
- Be a mentor, role model, administrator, and any other role necessary to educate students.

There is not one ingredient, there are numerous ingredients in the making of a successful instructor (Figure 3-1). Like any recipe, a good dish takes time to cook. It takes time for instructors to learn their limitations. The end product is an instructor who has become a seasoned, experienced, and motivational leader within the classroom.

This chapter looks at how to make this recipe. The ingredients are reviewed, emphasizing those characteristics used by successful instructors as well as characteristics that should be avoided, and why. In addition, some

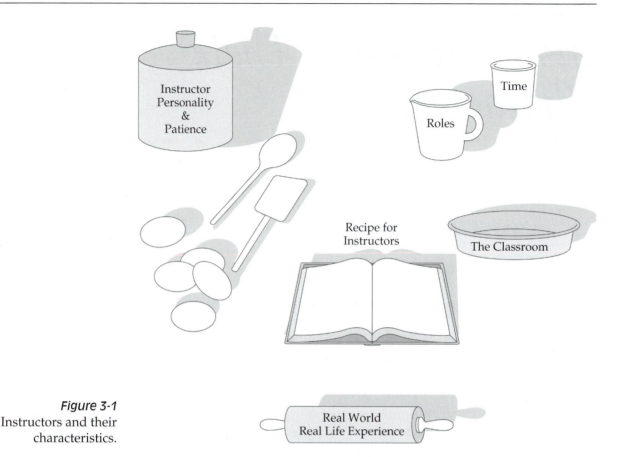

Figure 3-1
Instructors and their
characteristics.

of the fundamental techniques that allow instructors to better communicate with the students are discussed. Finally, there are techniques that can assist an instructor to improve the lesson presentation. But, first, let's discuss the definitions of *instruction* and *instructors*.

Instruction and Instructors

These two terms are used to define specific educational aspects of a training program. To understand the teaching process, a working definition of both terms must be identified.

Webster's New World Dictionary defines *instruction* as "to communicate knowledge, to teach." This definition can be refined to:

> *Instruction is the educational process that causes a student to learn material. This is also known as causing a change in the student's behavior.*

The goal of "causing a change in the student's behavior" is a primary educational principle. Changing the student's behavior is a working definition for learning. The entire educational process is planned and implemented around changing the student's behavior. Understanding the concept and definition of instruction will assist an instructor to understand the educational process.

The definition of *instructor* is related to instruction. An instructor's main job is to provide students with the experiences that will change their behavior. How an instructor accomplishes this job is the subject of the remainder of this chapter.

Motivation

To learn, a student must be stimulated by the subject. Motivating a student becomes a primary goal of instruction, that is, *motivation = learning.* Thus the instructor incorporates not only factual material but includes a variety of motivational techniques in order to stimulate the learning process.

But how much motivation is required to cause a change in a student's behavior? Unfortunately, there is no easy answer to this question. Part of the answer lies within an educational debate, a debate that concerns two teaching principles, the art and science of teaching. As you will see, this debate is deeply rooted in several educational philosophies.

There are degrees of influence that "the art of teaching" (idealism) and "the science of teaching" (realism) have upon the learning process. The art of teaching deals with the personality traits that an instructor incorporates into a lesson. The science of teaching is concerned with the planning, use, and evaluation of material contained within a lesson. Many instructors may be quick to note that anyone can design a lesson plan, but it takes a crafted instructor to teach the material. Conversely, a lesson must contain material. It is the degree of material that is presented that influences the learning process. A key factor in the debate deals with the personality characteristics of the instructor. If the instructor is dynamic, outgoing, and charismatic, the lesson tends to be taught using the "individualistic" approach, rather than the scientific approach. The instructor's personality characteristics provide the motivation within the lesson. Motivational techniques are not just based upon the art of teaching. The use of audiovisual aids, teaching strategies, teaching methods, and even the classroom facilities are considered motivational factors. How an instructor uses these motivational approaches is dependent upon the personality traits of the instructor. The next section addresses some of the personality characteristics associated with instructors.

Instructor Characteristics

The previous section identified the importance of the instructor's personality. Anyone can write a lesson plan, develop lesson materials, and prepare written examinations. The "teaching" part of the lesson is formed by the personality characteristics of the instructor.

The foremost characteristic is to "be yourself." Good instructors must identify their personal limitations. Not every teaching strategy, or teaching method, is designed for every instructor to use. Some instructors are fantastic lecturers, but have limited one-to-one teaching skills. Others are great at guided discussions and discovery methods of instruction, but feel constrained when placed in a lecture format (refer back to the science/art of

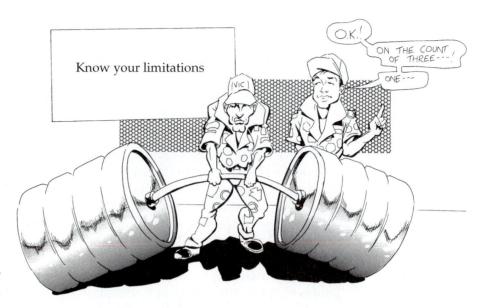

Know your
limitations.

teaching debate). In Chapter 2 a particularly useful personality assessment was identified. The Myers-Briggs assessment is a powerful assessment that instructors can use to identify their personality traits. Knowing these traits can help an instructor decide what instructional styles to use. Successful instructors identify teaching techniques that make them feel comfortable. Using teaching approaches that make instructors feel comfortable helps them to teach within their capabilities.

Students are impressionable. First impressions lay the groundwork for the entire learning experience. If an instructor provides incorrect information, performs inaccurate demonstrations, or shows half-completed demonstrations, the impression left upon students is one that is less than "correct information." An instructor must be the role model for the students. An instructor is to provide correct information and demonstrations the first time they are presented. Students will follow the lead that is set by the instructor (Figure 3-2).

Students look at the instructor as the expert, that is, as the one who knows the information. Can instructors be knowledgeable in all aspects of a subject? Realistically, the answer is no. An instructor must know the basics of a subject. What is important is for instructors to know where to look for the information they need for a presentation. Firsthand knowledge and experience are great for an instructor to possess. It should be noted that instructors who have firsthand experience tend to have more confidence regarding the subject than instructors who lack the firsthand experience. Having firsthand experience is a requirement in classes that require high levels of safety and experience. Programs such as high-angle rescue, scuba diving, interior firefighting, or vehicle rescue are examples of programs in which instructors and their assistant instructors must be experts. Hanging off a building, ten stories up, is not the place to find out that this is the instructor's first time to demonstrate a rescue scenario. Not every emergency service training program requires a high level of firsthand expertise. In-

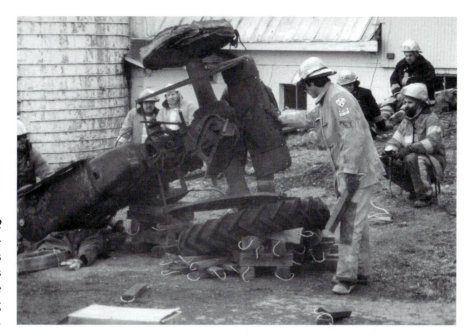

Figure 3-2
Students can get injured. Instructors must be experts when students are in threatening situations.

structors need to know the presentation material, and knowing the material does not always mean that they have to have firsthand experience.

Being yourself, being a role model, and being the expert are essential traits that instructors must exhibit. Without knowing their ability and being able to present the information safely and correctly, any other instructional characteristic is meaningless.

One way to become a successful instructor is to follow the footsteps that have been made by other instructors. Take a minute to think about the following question:

> *Throughout your formal education, you have met a dynamic and unique instructor. It could have been in high school, college, technical training school, or an emergency service training program. This individual found the right formula to motivate you to learn the material. What characteristics, or approaches, did that instructor use?*

The following list[1] identifies positive instructor characteristics. There is no priority to the listing. Chances are, some of your answers will appear on this list:

- Is well prepared
- Is knowledgeable
- Is flexible
- Cannot wait to go to class
- Exudes enthusiasm; is fun to be with

---

[1]This list and the list of "don't characteristics" are compiled from several years of comments generated from instructors answering the questions. What is surprising is the regularity of responses between the groups of instructors.

- Uses appropriate body language
- Makes eye contact with students
- Uses a variety of voice inflections
- Exhibits respect for students
- Utilizes innovative teaching methods
- Employs humor during presentations
- Is punctual with lesson presentations
- Moves throughout the classroom
- Reinforces and provides positive feedback to students
- Maintains a steady pace for the presentation
- Dresses appropriately for the class
- Says nothing, pauses, instead of saying "uh" or "um"
- Varies vocabulary to fit the students
- Encourages student participation
- Brings realism to presentations
- Supplements lesson material with varied and appropriate audio-visual aids
- Displays a professional demeanor
- Makes a relaxed presentation
- Stresses personal safety and watches out for the students
- Is caring and has compassion for the students
- Is likable
- Is honest and admits when an error occurs or admits "I don't know the answer"
- Is prepared for the unexpected; remembers "Murphy's law"
- Stays calm and rational
- Remembers the phrase, "Being yourself"

Write in your special instructor's characteristics:

- _____
- _____
- _____

The list ends with "being yourself," the importance of which cannot be overstated. Many more characteristics and techniques can be added to this list. But the making of an instructor comes from within each individual. Successful instructors use teaching approaches that make their presentations "theirs" and not someone else's. Add your answers to the list and remember these characteristics when you are "the instructor."

THE DON'T CHARACTERISTICS

The easy way to list the "don't characteristics" is to simply add *not* or *does not* in front of each of the positive characteristics. There are specific "do not's" that also need to be identified.

You are now back in your schooling experience. You are now in the worst class you have ever taken. The instructor is absolutely the worst

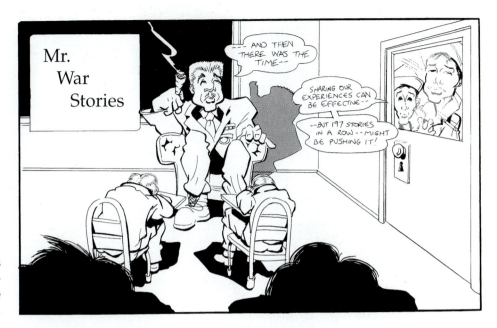

Mr. War Stories has no place in emergency service classrooms.

you have ever had. What did the instructor do to create such a poor learning experience?

The following list may contain some of your comments, but before you read on, STOP! Compare this list to the previous list. Ask yourself these questions:

- Does one list have more comments than the other?
- Was it easier to identify the negative comments or the positive comments?

Chances are, it probably was easier to identify the negative comments, and the negative list was probably as long or longer than the positive list. This is commonly seen when making these types of comparisons. Instructors must learn to balance both the positive and negative aspects of a student's performance and to limit their desire to focus on the negative aspects of a student's performance (Figure 3-3). Having said this, let's look at your answers and compare them to the following list. These characteristics are not inclusive and are not prioritized:

- Is inflexible
- Is not fun
- Yells at students who perform incorrectly
- Avoids direct eye contact with students
- Ignores concerns for student safety
- Motivates students by threats and failure
- Presents a poorly prepared lesson for the class
- Reads directly from a textbook to conduct the lesson
- Encourages off-colored humor or sexist comments
- Fails to have concern for the student's best interests
- Belittles students

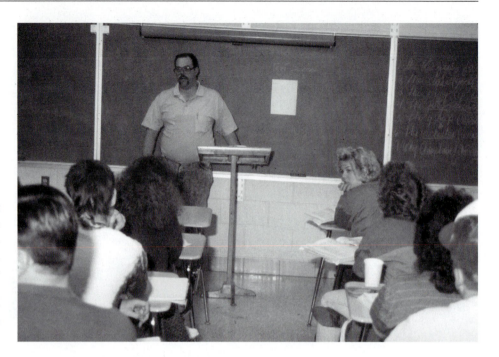

Figure 3-3
Balancing positive and negative comments or criticisms is a key responsibility for an instructor. Don't get tied up looking at just one side all the time.

- Does not communicate information effectively
- Relates "war stories" and displays a superior attitude to the students
- Is late for the class
- Consumes alcohol before or during a presentation
- Uses terms beyond the level of the students
- Stands in one place for the entire lesson
- Reads the lesson from notes
- Twirls slide remote or plays with chalk, pens, and the like
- Uses teaching approaches not within the personality of the instructor—those that are not their own

Write in your answers.

- _____
- _____
- _____

If a teaching approach feels uncomfortable, it probably is a "don't characteristic." These characteristics create a less than effective learning experience. If a teaching method or personality charactistic negatively affects a student learning experience, it becomes a don't characteristic and should be avoided.

Both lists are ingredients that form an instructor. Like any recipe, good ingredients make a quality product. Ingredients need the right mixing to make the recipe complete. The next section looks at the mixing component of the recipe, the instructor's roles.

Instructor Roles

An instructor has to wear multiple hats—"roles"—when instructing. Knowing when to wear the right hat influences the learning experience. Three instructor roles/characteristics have already been identified, "being yourself," "being a role model," and "being the expert." Let's look at some other instructor roles.

Instructors use a variety of roles to encourage, motivate, evaluate, and often discipline students. Some instructor roles end up having little benefit and can be harmful. In their book *Educational Psychology: A Realistic Approach*,[2] Thomas Good and Jere Brophy identify dominant instructor roles:

1. *Taskmaster:* Sets clear standards of performance for the students to attain. Supervises all student activity. Lessons are specifically identified and little deviation occurs within the lesson.
2. *Salesperson:* Stresses the importance of all program information. Every detail is important and is useful to the students, if not now, then later on. The lessons are taught from the perspective that if it is in the curriculum, it must be taught.
3. *Cheerleader:* Sells the personality and friendship of the instructor to the students. The instructor encourages and provides only positive reinforcement to students. Statements are sugarcoated and contain little constructive criticism.
4. *Carping Critic:* Insists that nothing that a student does is correct; there is always something wrong. Rarely is advice given to make corrective actions.
5. *Reality Therapist:* Tends to support the students to learn information at their own pace. Is supportive of any actions taken by the student. Provides encouragement and corrective action, as they are needed.

An instructor must be able to switch between the roles, depending on the learning situation. For example, if a student is having difficulty with a skill, the reality therapist role may provide the best support, whereas the taskmaster or the carping critic would be destructive.

Aside from the instructor roles Good and Brophy identify, there are other characteristics that instructors use fluently throughout a presentation. The following are commonly used roles or characteristics:

- Mentor
- Program administrator
- Friend
- Facilitator or experiential moderator
- Peer
- Authoritarian or disciplinarian

---

[2]Jere Brophy and Thomas Good, *Educational Psychology: A Realistic Approach* (New York: Holt, Rinehart and Winston, 1977).

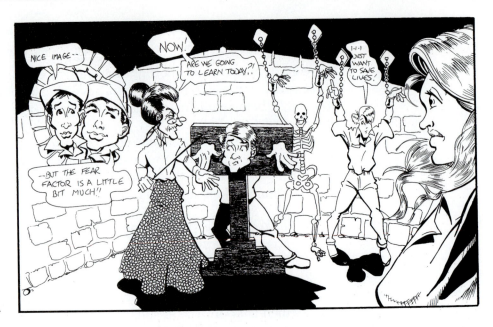

Taskmaster.

- Entertainer
- Judge or arbitrator
- Evaluator or examination designer
- Supervisor or manager
- Public relations specialist
- Logistical specialist
- Safety officer
- Resident expert in a topic or specialty
- Clerical staff
- Research analyst
- Equipment procurement and maintenance
- Any other role necessary to motivate and educate students

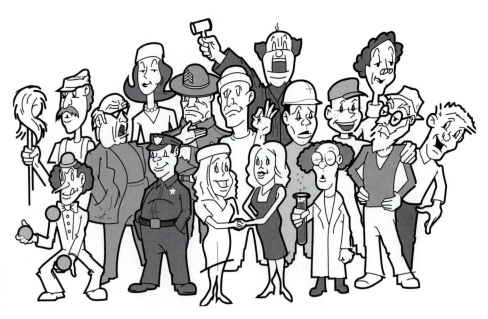

The diversified roles an instructor has in a classroom.

There is no specific ranking to these characteristics. Some are more important than others, like mentoring and being a facilitator. These two characteristics will be discussed further in this chapter in the section titled, "The Art of the Little Things." An instructor can be expected to use any or all of these characteristics. In the program administration chapter, a training institute's core structure is identified. The size and composition of the institute often dictate how many of these instructional roles or characteristics an instructor will be required to use. In most cases, it is the lesson topic, lesson plan, and students that will control which hat an instructor will need to wear.

The use of any role has its drawbacks. At best the instructor will stimulate and evaluate students honestly. But whatever tools are used, the instructor still has to teach the basics, or principles of instruction. Principles of instruction are the topic discussed in the next section.

Principles of Instruction

> *The teacher told us to use the tools this way, but when we went to the breakout station, the other instructor showed us another way. Which one is right? . . . Which one is the way I need to do it for the test? . . . I'm confused.*

Too often these types of comments are heard from students as they are going through the learning process. Their questions are valid. Their concerns are valid. And their confusion is real. So, how can an instructor deal with these issues? Is it the instructor's fault? The answer to these questions can be found within the concept of "principles of instruction." The principles of instruction can be seen in the following example.

A motto for vehicle rescue is that it is "the science of alternatives." There are many ways to open a damaged door. Each of the ways is correct, as long as they do not cause injury to the patient or to the rescuers. Thus the principle of instruction is to gain entry through the door without causing harm to the patient or to the rescuer. This task is accomplished by using any number of various methods.

Webster's New World Dictionary defines *principle* as "the ultimate source, origin, or cause of something" Using this definition, an instructor designs a lesson plan emphasizing the basic lesson material. Once a student understands the basic concepts, a variety of techniques can be used by the student to accomplish the lesson's objectives.

To identify the components associated with a principle, the instructor must

1. Examine the principle.
2. Identify the uses associated with the principle.
3. Determine methods that can be used with the principle.
4. Evaluate how the principle was used.

This evaluation process can be used to assess any principle. Accompanying this discussion is an example that everyone should be able to relate to—the use of a roll of paper towels (Figure 3-4). Sounds simple, but what is the

A Roll of Paper Towels
The Principle Is??

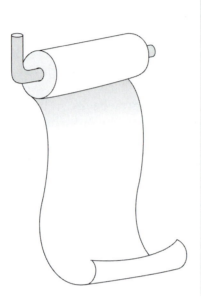

1. Examine the roll:
    • Size — Shape — Texture
    • Ideally designed for cleaning

2. Uses of the roll:
    • Cleaning — Strainer — Napkin
      and a 101 other uses!!!!

3. Methods for using the roll:
    • Rip a towel off and wipe mess up
    • Rip a towel off and lay out flat
      to use it as a placemat
    • etc....

4. Evaluate the towel:
    • Does it clean the mess up??
    • Does it work the first time???

Figure 3-4
Paper towel example.   The basic principle is for cleaning and it has a variety of other uses.

basic principle? What does a roll look like? How big is it? How can it be used? How can you use it? Does it work? Answer these questions, and you have found the principle. Try using the process on the following emergency service topics:

• A vacuum splint
• A spanner wrench
• A haligan bar

Using principles of instruction will lessen a student's confusion regarding a specific method of instruction. There may be a preferred way for accomplishing a task, but it is not the only way. Identifying the basics and teaching principles, not methods, is the recommended approach.

The Art of the Little Things

The lesson plan is written, student activities are planned, the examinations are written, the logistics (training equipment, assistant instructors, support equipment, etc.) have been taken care of, and the instructor has reviewed the lesson material. But is the instructor really ready? Is there something missing? Quite possibly there are—"the little things."

These little things encompass a wide variety of personal mannerisms, or "touches," that make a program special. Let's examine some of these special touches.

Talk to the Students   Prior to the class, during breaks, and after the class, spend time with the students. Getting to know the students' perspective allows the instructor to better relate the lesson material during the presentation. More important, it shows the students that you are not unreachable and are open to discussion. It shows you care about what the students have to say. This is where the "friend" instructor role is used!

Prepare Handout Material   Instructors pull resources from various sources to create a lesson plan. Handout materials often are copied from magazines, journals, notes, or other resource materials. Each may have a different font style, page number, and clarity. To improve the handout materials, spend some time to place the material in a standard font style. Then have the handout material numbered sequentially, so you and the students can easily reference the material. Last, place the material in a binder or a folder. These techniques help make your presentation appear more professional.

Bring Realism to the Presentation   Chapter 2 outlined a key adult learner trait: adults need realism. Expand upon this need and make the presentation as realistic as possible, even if this means bringing in experts, going on field trips, using computer simulations, setting up a satellite teleconference, using creative makeup techniques, or reviewing actual case studies to make a presentation come alive (Figure 3-5). More ideas are discussed in Chapter 13.

Razzle-Dazzle the Students   Linked with the previous item, as part of motivating the students, adults want to be impressed. Pull out the "bag of tricks" occasionally. Use multimedia presentations to spruce up a dull subject. Create a game to involve the students in the learning process. Contact a product vendor and have the newest equipment shown to the students.

Be a Caring Instructor   Students bring a host of personal problems into the classroom. Be understanding to a student who is not performing to potential; there may be a very good reason. Listening to the student may help both you and the student understand why the student is performing poorly.

Body Language Is a Subject All by Itself   Identified in the instructor characteristics section of this chapter, body language is a "big little thing." Not looking at the students, not engaging in eye contact, or crossing your arms and appearing to have a stern look on your face when confronted by a student's question are examples that illustrate poor body language. Even if an instructor is truly sincere, the body language can give an entirely different message.

Body language can be controlled. But before poor body language can be corrected, the instructor must first recognize it. An excellent way to

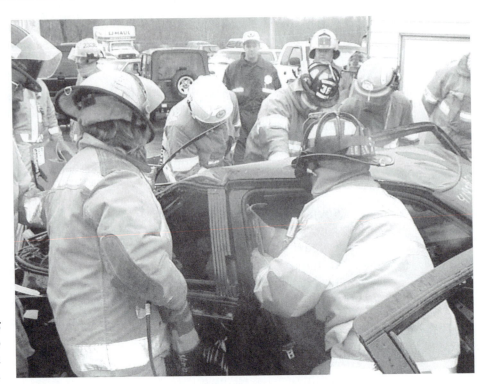

Figure 3-5
Do what it takes to
bring realism to a
presentation.

evaluate yourself as an instructor is to videotape your presentation. See the presentation from the student's perspective. Many instructors cannot believe what is taped. Not only body language, but the lesson delivery, classroom management skills, and student evaluation techniques can be evaluated using this approach. Only when instructors recognize their weaknesses can they make realistic changes to their body language or lesson presentation.

A Lesson's Perspective   In the film *The Dead Poets Society*, Robin Williams encouraged his students to develop and expand their thoughts, experiences, and knowledge. Each student was directed to rip out of his textbooks a written critique regarding a particular poem. Later, Williams had each student stand on top of the teacher's desk and look out across the classroom. He asked each student to see the classroom from a different perspective. He encouraged students not to just read a poem, but to express it and live out the poem.

This example shows an instructor who has not placed barriers in front of the students. He has encouraged the students to develop their knowledge and not to be happy with the basics. As instructors, expanding the student's perspective is a part of designing a quality training program. Part of the teacher's role is to provide opportunities for students to gain firsthand experience and then to draw their own conclusions. Teachers design their presentations to allow the students to express and live out their educational experiences. Seeing students living out their experiences is what makes being an instructor worthwhile.

Spice Up the Classroom   "Little surprises" often enable an instructor to motivate a class that is showing signs of being bored. There are a variety of tricks of the trade that seasoned instructors use to stimulate the students.

Reviewing the formula *motivation = learning,* the instructor's role is to be a motivator. Within this role, there can be a host of characters used to motivate students, so release a few of the characters by living out the personalities. If the topic is safety hazards, enter the classroom in the appropriate safety equipment—for example, SCBA, bunker gear, or latex gloves. If the topic is anatomy, locate a skeleton model and pick up different skeleton parts. Then carry them around the classroom during a class discussion. You might find that this will hold the students' attention, sort of like the eleven o'clock news briefs that stimulate your interest to tune in the news broadcast. Another approach is to hold a "special break session," where you bring in a vegetable tray or other "good" food snack one night out of the blue. Then while everyone is munching, hold an informal review session—a game of some sort is great in this type of environment. Do not be afraid to try something different, something out of the ordinary, or something that is just fun that motivates the students and reinforces learning.

Hook 'em the First Time   Students often judge a course by the way an instructor starts the lesson. If the introduction is bland and lifeless, chances are that many students will "turn off" their learning processes for that particular session. Professional performers say if you don't knock them dead in the first minute, you're done. Instruction is a little more forgiving. However, if you can "hook 'em" within the first five minutes of a presentation, you will have them for the rest of the program. Use some of the previous little things to further razzle-dazzle them. "Hook'em in the first five and you'll be alive!"

Dress for the Occasion   Identified in the listing of positive instructor traits, this "little thing" can affect a class's perception of the instructor (Figure 3-6). Coming into a fire department setting with a three-piece suit to make a presentation on hazardous environments is generally not the appropriate attire for the occasion. Conversely, presenting a prehospital topic to a group of nurses and physicians wearing blue jeans, a baseball hat, and a tee shirt with some trade-related slogan plastered over the entire front of the shirt is not appropriate either. Dressing for the occasion goes back to a concept covered in Chapter 2, get to know your audience. Find out the course location and who is attending your presentation. Being inappropriately dressed for a presentation sends the wrong message to the students. So make sure to "dress for the occasion" before leaving to teach.

Get to Know the Names of the Students and Call on Them by Name   It is inappropriate to say "hey, you" during the last week of a three-month program just because you have not gotten to know the student's name. Getting to know all the students, especially in large courses, may be something of a challenge, but it shows that the instructor cares about every student and values the student's comments.

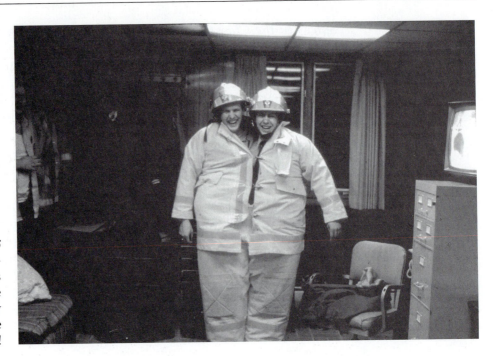

Figure 3-6
Team teaching protective clothing was on the minds of these two instructors. They were dressed for the occasion!

Use Analogies   Students may not understand new material because they have no frame of reference to which to compare it. Offering an analogy sometimes helps. For example, a challenging concept to teach in an emergency medical technician (EMT) course is that of shock. Many instructors have found that using a boiler plant to explain what happens in shock helps the students understand its effect in a human being (Figure 3-7).

Another analogy that can be used to explain a shock state is related to a fire engine and firehoses. Different hose sizes carry different amounts of volume and pressure. If a hose springs a leak, there will be a decrease in the volume and pressure in the hose. If the leak is not corrected, there will be a further loss of volume and pressure until the engine speed is increased to compensate the loss. The first line that the human body uses is for the heart to increase the rate to compensate the loss of volume (Figure 3-8).

An analogy is a powerful tool that instructors should use whenever possible. It makes a presentation come to life and will bring a new level of understanding to the classroom.

Be a Mentor   The ultimate positive experience instructors can create is having students excel by studying under their tutorship. This requires a significant commitment of time, patience, and support by both the instructor and the student. Mentoring is usually done in small groups on a one-to-one basis. The instructor shares in-depth knowledge of a subject and assigns students tasks that challenge their intellectual and physical abilities. Not every student and instructor is cut out to participate in a mentoring program. It also does not have to be a mentoring program between the instructor and students. Mentoring can be done between students, previous students, or assistant instructors. As students talk about a subject and gain an awareness of the material, the end result will be an improvement in their

Analogy for a hypovolemic shock condition

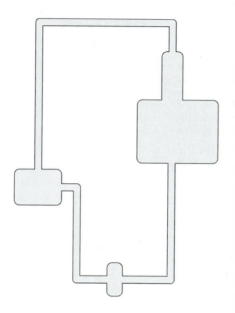

A Boiler Plant

1. Boiler
2. Pipes
3. Regulators

If the system develops a leak, the entire boiler system will experience a decrease in pressure. The regulators will have the boiler turn on to try to increase the pressure. Eventually the system will fail when the water volume is depleted.

The human body has a pump (the heart), pipes (the arteries and veins), and regulators (the brain). Without blood in the system, it too will fail (shock).

Figure 3-7
Analogy for a hypovolemic shock condition.

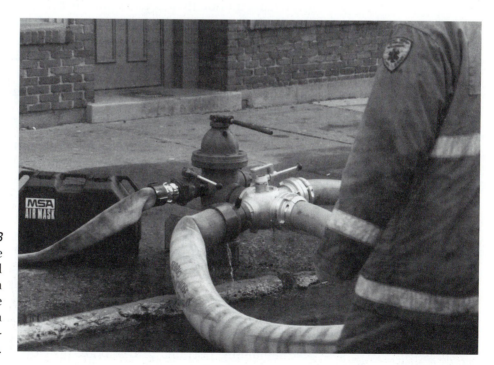

Figure 3-8
A leak in a firehose causes a volume and pressure loss. In a human, a leak in the circulatory system causes a drop in volume and pressure.

retention of the information. Challenge yourself and your students to excel; mentoring works!

Be a Facilitator   The pragmatic's view of instruction is that an instructor should be a facilitator of information exchange. In the next chapter, John Dewey's pragmatic educational philosophy is discussed in depth. The students should actively participate in the lesson presentation. The instructor should help guide the students to the lesson's objectives, while letting the students reach their own conclusions. Being a facilitator is a vital role instructors use when using the experiential learning model. Instructors do not have to be the sole lecturer. Being a facilitator is a fulfilling role for both the instructor and students.

Show Passion   The last art of the little things is passion. Passion, as it is used here, is the commitment and motivation an instructor shows when teaching. Passionate instructors approach teaching with a "fire," "attitude," an "intensity" and "commitment," and a "love for the art of teaching"—instructional chutzpa!

Summary

Want to become a successful instructor? Well, a simple approach would be to adopt the positive instructor traits outlined in this chapter. However, in real life, events do not always allow for the best performance. Instructors are not superior beings; instructors make mistakes and are not always able to perform to the best of their ability. In these cases, be responsible, admit an error has been made, and move on. Striving to be a competent instructor becomes a motivator for the instructor. An instructor who is motivated approaches instructing with passion and transfers this energy to the students.

Motivation = learning, which leads to an enriched learning environment.

It would be nice to have an all-encompassing recipe for becoming a successful instructor. Unfortunately, there is no such thing. Of the essential instructor characteristics listed, the most important trait is to be yourself. Trying to accomplish tasks beyond the reach of an instructor's ability is counterproductive. Using methods of instruction that feel comfortable is essential.

Start becoming a good instructor by being yourself and use only those characteristics that will allow your students to experience the material by being actively involved in the learning process.

The opening recipe provides insights into the making of a successful instructor. This chapter has only just begun to explore all the characteristics that make an instructor. For any one of the traits, there may be an entire chapter. Instructors who are able to marry their knowledge, experience, personality, compassion, and the desire to share these characteristics with students become successful instructors.

The remaining portions of this book provide the tools to become a successful instructor. From teaching strategies, to teaching methods, to the various evaluation tools, each will enhance the quality of a presentation.

Chapter 4

Theories and Concepts of Education

➤ OBJECTIVES

- Assess and review key educators and their learning theories.
- Identify how historic learning theories have shaped today's educational system.
- Identify the learning theories associated with cognitive learning.
- Identify and discuss the influence of various educational philosophies. Specific philosophies reviewed include:
  —Idealism
  —Realism
  —Humanism (Perennialism)
  —Essentialism
  —Pragmatism (Progressivism)
  —Behaviorism
  —Reconstructionism
- Identify how students learn.

To understand where we have been points us ahead to where we want to be. Reviewing history from this perspective allows today's education to benefit from previous years of experience.

The instructional methods in today's classroom did not just appear; they are the result of years of educational research. Theories and educational philosophies influence today's emergency service classrooms.

Educational history reveals a who's who list of educational leaders. Ivan Pavlov, E. L. Thorndike, B. F. Skinner, and John Dewey have contributed to today's educational system. Learning theories and educational philosophies can be associated with these historical individuals.

Why is it important to know the history and learning theories of education? Reread the opening quotation of this chapter, as the answer is contained within the quotation. Chapter 3 explained that instructors need to find out who they are and stay focused on their beliefs and abilities. As an instructor, you will find a particular education philosophy that you have already adopted as yours. In this chapter, as you read each educational theory and philosophy, try to identify which one reflects your beliefs. You will likely find that you use a hybrid of philosophies.

Behavioral Theories

In this section, we will look at theories that deal with learning through behavioral reinforcement. The theories noted in this section have evolved over several hundred years of research.

Classical Learning Theory   Ivan Pavlov and E. L. Thorndike are noted for pioneering the testing of classical learning theories. Pavlov's famous dog salivation experiments concluded that a learner can be conditioned to respond to specific stimuli. Thorndike built upon Pavlov's theories in his work with the concept of "trial and error." He determined that a learner needed to be motivated to solve a problem.[1]

Stimulus-Response Theory   E. R. Guthrie refined the classical conditioning approaches and contributed to "stimulus–response" theory.[2] The theory said that for every stimulus there is a corresponding response. He found that learning could occur during the first contact with a stimulus and that complete learning could occur. But usually, continued reinforcement was required to retain the information.

Task Analysis Theory   R. M. Gagne developed the task analysis theory.[3] He looked at a task (specifically useful to determine skills) and broke the task into various components. For skill development, an instructor needs to use positive reinforcement, especially when a skill is initially learned (Figure 4-1). Questions that are commonly asked in a task analysis include:

> What is important to learning?
> What is essential to learning?
> What makes the learning task difficult/easy?

From these questions, an instructor's lesson plan can better relate the information to the students.

Reinforcement (S-R) Theory   B. F. Skinner is noted for his work in partial reinforcement habits (reinforcement theory). His work centered on defining specific responses to stimuli. The concept of behavioral shaping is associated with Skinner. The reinforcement theory identifies how an instructor can influence how students learn. Positive reinforcement is the key to successful learning. Behaviors that are positively reinforced are likely to be repeated.

It is important to note that any form of reinforcement, positive or negative is needed. Students need to have a "Knowledge of Results" **(KR)** to learn. Even negative feedback is better than no feedback. With no feedback,

---

[1]Jere Brophy and Thomas Good, *Educational Psychology: A Realistic Approach* (New York: Holt, Rinehart and Winston, 1977).

[2]E. Guthrie, *The Psychology of Learning* (New York: Harper and Brothers, 1952).

[3]R. Gagne and L. Briggs, *Principles of Instructional Design* (New York: Holt, Rinehart and Winston, 1974).

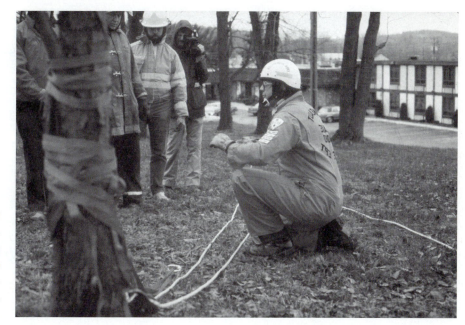

Figure 4-1
For skill development, an instructor needs to use positive reinforcement, especially when a skill is initially learned.

students develop a "numb" response. These students assume that no feedback must mean that what they are learning is satisfactory, or that it just does not matter to the instructor if learning is occurring. Learning must be accomplished through KR and instructors must be the facilitators of KR.

Cognitive Theories

Cognitive theories stress the use of mental capabilities. Learning is influenced by the individual's ability to think and discover information. Cognitive educators have students discover information rather than rely upon the instructor to provide the information (Figure 4-2). Students are encouraged to become active processors of information.

One of the fundamental cognitive theories is the **Gestalt theory.**[4] This theory looks at how students group information and react to that information. Perception and problem-solving skills are extensively used in this theory.

Jean Piaget is considered one of the principle researchers associated with the cognitive learning principles.[5] In one of Piaget's research studies, he discovered that small children respond differently to questions than older children because of their perceptions of the information. Much of his research was centered on how individuals perceive and react to the information.

---

[4]W. D. Ellis, *A Source Book of Gestalt Psychology* (New York: Harcourt, Brace & World, 1938).

[5]Jean Piaget, *The Child's Conception of the World* (New York: Littlefield Adams, 1990).

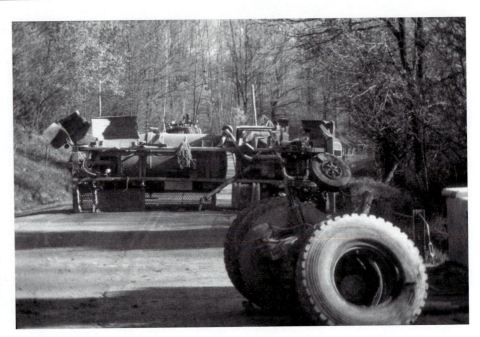

Figure 4-2
Cognitive thinking plays a crucial role in the size-up of a vehicle accident.

In Chapter 2, David Kolb's learning style inventory was discussed.[6] The LSI inventory is actually based on cognitive theory concepts. When learners are learning information, they process (i.e., "perceive") information based on their learning style preference.

"Right Brain and Left Brain Thinking" theory is based on medical and psychological research.[7] Our brain consists of two hemispheres, the right and left sides. Each side of the brain controls different emotions and behaviors. These differences determine how individuals react to situations. In most cases, individuals will have a preferred side. "Left Brain" thinking tends to be objective, logical, and analytical. "Right Brain" thinking is subjective, creative, and is an emotional center. How a student or instructor reacts to a situation is based on which side of their brain they favor. What is the significance of this research? Instructors should plan lesson activities that challenge both types of thinkers.

Cognitive learning is an important part of emergency service training programs. Students must be able to perform "discovery" tasks. Consider, for instance, an automobile accident. EMS, fire, and rescue personnel must "discover" a safe but rapid extrication route to remove a critically injured victim from a wrecked automobile. These life and death decisions are made as the result of an individual being able to use cognitive learning skills. Students in emergency service training programs must be taught to think for

---

[6]David Kolb, *The Learning Style Inventory* (Boston: McBer, 1985).
[7]Bernice McCarthy, *The 4MAT System: Teaching to Learning Styles with Right/Left Mode Techniques* (Chicago, IL: Excel, Inc., 1980).

themselves. Our role as instructors is to provide students with the opportunity to explore and develop these thinking processes.

Facilitator Theories

Facilitation theories are relatively new, in comparison to the behavioral and cognitive theories. Simply, these theories recognize that students learn, retain, and have an enriched learning experience when they are actively involved in the learning process. These theories are creating new paradigms for the education system. Many of the facilitation theories are based on educational concepts pioneered by Piaget and Dewey. Facilitation theorists believe that instructors should be the conductors of information exchange and the students should be the orchestra for obtaining the information.

Constructivist Theory   In this theory, students construct their own knowledge by trying new ideas and approaches, based on their prior knowledge and experience.[8] Students then apply the new knowledge to new situations. Students are actively involved in the constructivist theory. Instructors design problem-solving activities that challenge the students. Students are encouraged not to memorize information but instead to form an understanding of the information based on their experiences.

Instructors face unique challenges in teaching this theory.[9] The constructivist instructor must design program activities around the student's prior knowledge. Instructors use freewheeling discussions, simulations, and various problem-solving activities to encourage students to analyze and evaluate the information. The instructor is the facilitator and encourages students to think beyond traditional information.

Experiential Learning Theory   According to John Dewey, "Experience is the best teacher; in the final analysis the direct experience may be the only dependable teacher. . . . people do not want to be taught, they want to learn. . . . the best way to learn is through experience."[10] Students learn information by reflecting on their past experiences.[11] The learning experience is designed around the needs of the learner. The instructor uses role-playing, problem solving, group discussions, and self-reflection activities to allow students to discover information on their own terms.

---

[8]J. Bruner, *Going Beyond the Information Given* (New York: Norton, 1973).

[9]C. M. Reigeluth, "A new paradigm of ISD?" *Educational Technology,* May-June 1996, 13–20.

[10]John Dewey, *Democracy and Education: An Introduction to the Philosophy of Education* (New York: Macmillan, 1930).

[11]David A. Kolb, *Experiential Learning: Experience as the Source of Learning and Development* (Upper Saddle River, N.J.: Prentice Hall, 1984); C. R. Rogers, *Freedom to Learn* (Columbus, Ohio: Merrill/Macmillan, 1969); C. R. Rogers and H. J. Freiberg, *Freedom to Learn,* 3rd ed. (Columbus, Ohio: Merrill/Macmillan, 1994).

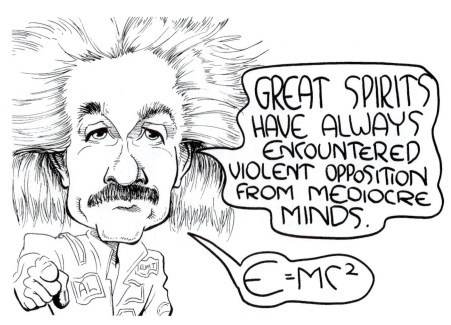

Courtesy of the Baker St. Group.

Learning theories play a vital role in the development of educational programming for emergency service training programs. Based on these theories are the educational philosophies discussed next.

Educational Philosophies

What type of instructor are you going to be? Whenever you start thinking about what kind of instructor you will be, the educational philosophies that you believe in will guide you to the answer. This section looks at the philosophies of education.[12] Emphasis has been placed upon the effects of the philosophy on an instructor. Think about each philosophy and make a judgment on how it matches your beliefs.

Idealism   Instructors in this philosophy tend to be highly personalized, creative, and individualized. They encourage the "art of teaching." They like dealing with people. These instructors encourage a freedom of individual expression. Their liberal approach centers on the students. Discussion and open discussion formats are the preferred approaches. The goal of an idealist is to educate students rather than spoon-feed the information to the students, in essence training the students.

---

[12]Don-chea Chu, *Philosophic Foundations of American Education* (Dubuque, Iowa: Kendall/Hunt, 1971); John D. Pullman, *History of Education in America*, 2nd ed. (New York: Macmillan, 1987); John Dewey, *Democracy and Education: An Introduction to the Philosophy of Education* (New York: Macmillan, 1930); *Pennsylvania Department of Health Rescue Instructor Curriculum* (Harrisburg: The Department, 1983); Jere Brophy and Thomas Good, *Educational Psychology: A Realistic Approach* (New York: Holt, Rinehart and Winston, 1977); David Kolb, *Learning Style Inventory* (Boston: McBer, 1985).

Realism   An opposite perspective to idealism is a realistic instructor who stresses a scientific approach. Classes have structure. Instructors tend to be machinelike, factual, and objective; to encourage a mastery of factual information; and to be the providers of the information.

A realistic instructor loves to teach through the use of lectures and structured demonstrations. The "systematic approach" to instruction is the way a lesson is delivered. In the systematic approach, an instructor prepares, presents, and evaluates. The realistic instructor's main concern is to measure how much information was learned, not to see if the student attained an education.

Instructors feel that they are the specialist or expert. Their main role is to provide the information and then to tell the students the conclusions that they should reach. This type of approach is also known as the inductive approach to learning. The instructor does the work while the students are asked to show up and listen.

Humanism (perennialism)   This philosophy can be called "the discipline of the mind." The instructor encourages each student to be self-motivated and to gain an understanding of the information through mental experience. Abstract thinking and using a student's imagination are key assets.

Students are encouraged to think for themselves. There is little structure to this form of teaching. Instructors set few or no barriers, and the class is taught through open discussion and work groups. Instructors believe that the more a student can think about the information and solve problems on his own, the better the educational experience. Open, freewheeling discussions involve both the instructor and students. Together issues are debated and a holistic viewpoint is reached.

Essentialism   Called "educational conservationists," these instructors believe that if the information is not immediately important, then it does not need to be taught. This approach is very logical, while being very rigid at the same time. Solid learning is stressed rather than entertainment. Students need the basic information, not a lot of "it's nice to know" type of information.

Instructors deliver information without a lot of thrills. Students are attending the program to learn information. Lectures, few individual learning experiences, and a strict compliance to "the standards" are the main teaching approaches. A return to the basics of knowledge and skills is the goal of an essentialism instructor.

Pragmatism (progressivism)   The pragmatic approach is identified with John Dewey, an educator noted for the concept of "learning by doing." According to Dewey, "people do not want to be taught, they want to learn. . . . the best way to learn is through experience."[13] The pragmatism movement stresses the need for students to be given an opportunity to learn the

---

[13]John Dewey, *Democracy and Education: An Introduction to the Philosophy of Education* (New York: Macmillan, 1930).

information by experiencing it (Figure 4-3). Both art and science of instruction are joined together. Students must be able to observe and then be given an opportunity to participate.

Several specific learning theories are associated with the pragmatism approach. These include the following:

1. *Theory of relativism:* Nothing remains static or constant.
2. *Theory of practium:* Paying attention to the present.
3. *Theory of organicism:* Ideas are in process, progress, or making.

Instructors allow the students to solve realistic problems through realistic approaches whenever possible. Current events, classroom freedom, individualism, and actual life experiences are controlled through an experience centered curriculum. Instructors design programming that is controlled but allow students to experience the information (e.g., "Here's a power hydraulic tool. Identify different ways to remove a damaged door, keeping in mind safety concerns for the patient and for the rescuers"). Pragmatic instructors believe that knowledge is derived from experience. An instructor must provide the stimulus to make knowledge an active learning experience. Teaching approaches include discussion groups, field trips, audiovisual aids, interactive lab sessions, and demonstrations designed to elicit questions from the students. The lecture format is used, but only to provide basic information. The more a student can participate, the better.

Behaviorism   B. F. Skinner, J. Watson, and Ivan Pavlov are associated with this philosophy. Behaviorists believe that students respond to learning situations based on their external environment. Provide a student with positive or negative feedback and there will be a corresponding reaction.

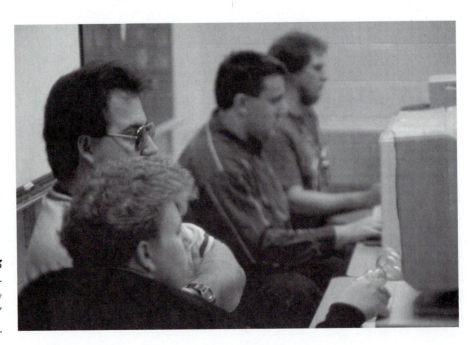

Figure 4-3
A learning experience is enhanced by students "doing" rather than listening.

Assure the learning environment is comfortable and provide positive feedback to the students and the result will be a student learning and retaining the information.

Instructors must provide students with a positive learning environment: Clean and well lit classrooms, comfortable chairs, up-to-date presentation materials, and positive feedback interactions by the instructional staff. Positive reinforcement must be stressed at every learning opportunity.

Reconstructionism In the reconstructionism philosophy, a teacher becomes a coordinator of information. The presentations are taught based upon the needs of the students. Specific goals are set and the lesson is developed around the needs of the students. The lesson is flexible and is driven by the goals that are set for the group of students.

Students must be highly motivated and must want to learn the information. The instructor encourages the students to look at the whole learning experience. Self-thinking and rationalizations are encouraged. The students are learning for a specific purpose rather than learning general information for multiple purposes.

Overview of Philosophies

Which philosophy do you feel describes your teaching style? Are you an instructor who teaches by the "art" of teaching or are you more concerned with the content of the lesson? Will you encourage students to think about the information or do you want them to learn enough information to accomplish the lesson assignment? Or do you want them to learn by doing?

All are interesting approaches to teaching students. Instructors tend to favor one philosophy and then mix other philosophies into their lesson presentation. The instructor's personality becomes a determinant in the selection of the philosophy that the instructor uses. The group of students that is being taught also becomes an additional determinant. Students who have a practical orientation would be taught better using the pragmatic approach rather than the humanistic approach. As noted in Chapter 2, an instructor needs to know who the students are and adapt the lesson plan to the type of students being taught.

Emergency service training programs have been influenced by all the philosophies of education. A training institute, an instructor, or the students can play a role in determining the use of a particular philosophy. Matching the philosophy with the teaching approach that is best suited for the students is an important aspect that cannot be overstated. This is where the historic philosophies of education impact today's emergency service classes.

WHAT'S YOUR PHILOSOPHY?

You have reviewed the theories and philosophies. What is your educational philosophy? Insert the CD-ROM and click on Philosophy Assessment. The assessment is designed to assess your dominant philosophies.

What Is Learning?

A dictionary definition of learning says that learning is the attaining of knowledge or a skill about a specific subject or process. Instructors are concerned whether or not learning has occurred. So far, Chapters 2 and 3 state factors and techniques that influence learning. But what is learning, beyond quoting a dictionary definition? Can we see learning occurring in our students? How do we learn? All are important questions.

The first characteristic that makes learning difficult to define is that it is invisible. An instructor cannot look at a student and see if the student is learning. Learning is a mental process. Students use human senses to attain the information. Then they associate the information with a previous experience. This association is important for remembering the information. An instructor knows if a student has learned the information only by observing their actions (behavior). When a change in behavior is noted by the instructor (e.g., a student is able to identify and use the padded board splints to immobilize a fractured elbow and was not able to do so before the lesson), an instructor can evaluate the amount of learning that has taken place. Creating a change in behavior is what the instructor's goal is in the teaching process.

HOW STUDENTS LEARN AND RETAIN INFORMATION

Educators have studied how students learn and retain information. Students can learn information through all the human senses. Exhibit 4-1 shows the percentage of learning that occurs through each of the senses; it also shows how students retain information using various stimuli.

Exhibit 4-1 has obvious implications for an instructor. In the first column, an instructor needs to have the students use their senses during every presentation: 94 percent of potential learning is accomplished through see-

Exhibit 4-1

Learning and Retention	
COLUMN 1	COLUMN 2
83% Learning by sight	10% Retention by reading
11% Learning by hearing	20% Retention by hearing
3% Learning by smell	30% Retention by sight
2% Learning by touch	50% Retention by sight and hearing
1% Learning by taste	70% Retention by talking
	90% Retention by doing

Permission granted by Anita J. Harrow, *A Taxonomy of the Psychomotor Domain: A Guide for Developing Behavioral Objectives* (New York: David McKay, 1972).

ing and hearing. Making each presentation stimulating depends upon the instructor's ability to plan events that make students use their senses.

The other senses, smell, touch, and taste, are more difficult to include in a lesson, but they are critical senses for emergency personnel. Take, for instance, a firefighter. It is important for an interior firefighter to be able to touch and feel for hot spots. Even more important, firefighters know that if they can smell smoke through the SCBA mask, they have a problem. These two senses are important to stress to students. A fire instructor builds lessons designed to stimulate these senses.

EMS instructors also key in on the senses of touch and smell. To assess a patient, a hands-on assessment is performed. Both senses are involved in this assessment. Grating of a broken bone or the identification of subcutaneous emphysema is made through touch. Often the assessment of a diabetic patient is made based upon an acetone smell. Other smells can be unpleasant, such as incontinence, burned skin, and emesis.

Emergency personnel do not frequently use the sense of taste. While some firefighters may argue that this sense is used to test "firemen's chili," in general, the sense of taste has little use in emergency training programs.

The retention chart shows that students may learn information but may not retain the information (Figure 4-4). As can be seen, reading a textbook provides only 10 percent retention of the information. An instructor who just talks can expect students to retain 20 percent of the information. In contrast, when an instructor uses audiovisual aids and encourages students' participation while providing the information, 70 percent of the information will be retained. The optimum retention, 90 percent or better, occurs by having the students directly experience the information.

Figure 4-4
The graph illustrates that learning and retention of information are related. The more senses that are stimulated increases the retention of information.

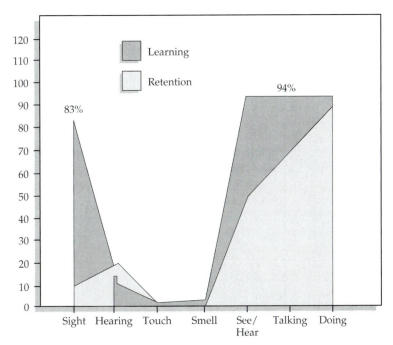

Learning and Retention

Learning and retaining information are linked. The graph illustrates this point. Using multiple senses increases the retention of information. Instructors need to design activities that stimulate a student's senses to increase the retention of the information. Do not forget the discussion from Chapter 3 regarding motivation; this is a graphic representation of the need for student–instructor motivation.

LEARNING SKILLS

A critical part of emergency service training programs is putting knowledge to work. Referred to as psychomotor development, students are shown how to physically use their knowledge, in other words to develop practical skills. Skill development is an active learning process, "learning by doing." As already noted, up to 90 percent retention of information occurs when students are actively involved in the learning experience. This section looks at how an instructor encourages students to become active learners.

Learning a skill takes time and practice to reach the 90 percent retention level. The learning curve for skill development shows that students develop skills in proportion to time (Figure 4-5). From the initial point to the mastery point, the improvement of a skill keeps rising until it reaches the mastery point, the goal for all students.

There are two development points between the initial and mastery levels, the plateau phase and the latency phase. Students often reach a point where they practice, but little skill improvement occurs. This plateau phase of learning often leads to another phase, the latency phase. Students make the same mistakes as they practice the skill over and over. Instructors must

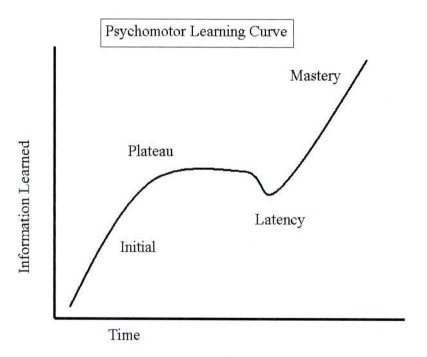

Figure 4-5
Skill learning curve. Four phases of skill development are the initial, plateau, latency, and mastery.

provide positive support to students in this phase. Often students do not realize that they are making a mistake. Videotaping the students performing the skill, coupled with reviewing the skill with the students, is helpful for these students to visualize their mistakes. Chapter 9 provides more detailed information for the development of skills. Information and skills are learned differently by each student. The next chapter looks at how a student learns information.

Summary

Think about the information that you just read. Were there any similarities between any theories, philosophies, and learning styles? The opening quote states that today's educational system is formed by its history. If you look at the theories, philosophies, and learning styles, a common thread runs through all of them. The theories are based on the philosophies, the philosophies are based on the theories, and the ways students learn information are based on both the philosophy and the theories.

In the beginning of this chapter, you were asked to find yourself as an instructor. One or more of the philosophies will become your dominant style. Your teaching style will be influenced by your personal learning style inventory. You will teach other students the way you learn information. David Kolb's learning style inventory is a powerful tool that instructors should use to assess who they are, so that they can better teach their students.

History and current research are affecting today's educational systems. Emergency service training programs have been and will be affected by new concepts and by old concepts. Knowing where we have been helps us to know where we need to be. Looking at the theories and philosophies that have shaped today's training programs is laying the foundation for tomorrow's educational system.

Chapter 5

Behavioral Objectives, Lesson Plans, and Curriculum

➤ OBJECTIVES

- Define *behavioral objective.*
- Identify the critical components of a behavioral objective:
  —Action (behavior)
  —Condition
  —Criteria (performance standards)
  —Audience (SWBAT or LWBAT)
- List acceptable action verbs for behavioral objectives.
- Identify behavioral objectives for cognitive, psychomotor, and affective domains.
- Describe the use of Bloom's *Taxonomy of Educational Objectives* for developing the behavioral objectives and lesson plan.
- Describe the use of Krathwohl's *Taxonomy of Educational Objectives, Handbook 2, Affective Domain.*
- Analyze how objectives affect the entire lesson plan, curriculum, and educational process.
- Describe the process used to develop and write behavioral objectives and a lesson plan.
- Identify how to create a lesson plan when using a standardized curriculum.
- Comment on the process used to evaluate a behavioral objective.
- Identify the essential components of a lesson plan.
- Identify different styles of lesson plans.
- State the uses and structure of lecture notes.
- Compare and contrast the use of a lesson plan and lecture notes.
- Identify the use of computers and computer software to design and use a lesson plan.
- Describe the development of a curriculum.
- Discuss noneducational uses of the lesson plan.

Instructional Architecture 101

The purpose of this chapter is to describe how to become a successful architect of lesson plan development and how to personalize standardized lesson plans. The majority of emergency services training programs use either standardized lesson plans or curricula. When using a standardized lesson presentation it needs to be created around the instructor's teaching style.

For example, EMS training programs and accrediting bodies use the U.S. DOT EMT Basic National Standard Curriculum (NSC) as the principle guideline for instructing and certifying EMT-B personnel throughout the United States. The EMT-B curriculum provides instructors with a lot of useful information. Included are behavioral objectives, a basic content outline, procedural information, student learning strategies, remediation and enrichment strategies, and evaluation concepts. The EMT-B curriculum is designed to establish a minimum educational standard. Accrediting agencies, training institutes, and instructors are to use the curriculum as a starting point for the instruction, certification, and establishment of the scope of practice for emergency medical personnel. It is up to the instructor and training institute to decide how to teach the curriculum.

So how is a curriculum designed? What goes into making a lesson plan? How does an instructor personalize a curriculum? The answers to these questions are contained in this chapter. To begin answering these questions, let's look at the following house building analogy.

A building contractor does not just go out and decide to build a house. The contractor consults an architect and together they design a blueprint for the house. Assembling the blueprint includes all the features that the homeowner wants in the house, plus ensuring its structural integrity, a floor plan for each room, a listing of supplies and materials, compliance with local building and inspection codes, and an estimate of the time to build the house. There are specific measurements for each room, specifications for the types of materials and supplies that are used, and a listing of subcontractors to do additional work in support of the general contractor. The contractor takes this blueprint and follows it to build the house.

The homeowner checks on the progress of the house as it is being built. Together with the contractor, corrections are made. Only when the house is completely built does the contractor receive his final payment.

Figure 5-1 is a blueprint for a lesson plan. Designing a lesson plan can be likened to designing a house; the components just have different titles. The behavioral objectives become the blueprints for the lesson's foundation and the standardized curriculum and scope of practice become the lesson plan's building codes. A lesson plan, like a house that is being built, requires a lot of planning, coordination of resources, technical knowledge and skill, and evaluation components. Knowing how to design, build, and use a lesson plan is an essential trait for an instructor.

Before Designing the Lesson

Before a lesson plan is designed, a working knowledge of "who the students are" (Chapter 2) and "who the instructors are" (Chapters 3 and 4) is vital. With an understanding of this information an instructor can prepare a lesson plan to meet the needs of the students, instructor, and the training institute.

Who the students are can be assessed by using a questionnaire. Determining the reading level of students is a little more difficult. Instructors tend to use a variety of methods for assessing the reading level of students. Methods range from their best guess, based on previous student perfor-

Blueprint for building a lesson plan

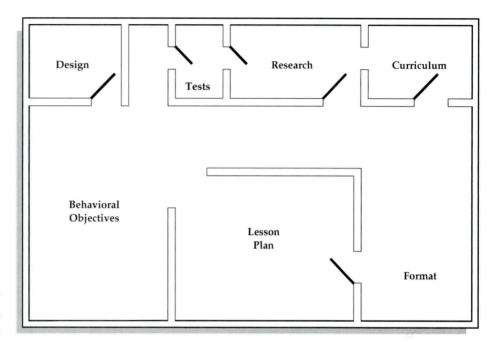

Figure 5-1
A lesson plan
blueprint.

mance, to a formal literacy entrance examination used to determine the reading level for a specific group of students, to a process that uses both options. Based on this information, behavioral objectives, the lesson plan, course materials, examinations, and the textbooks are selected, so that they meet the reading level of the students (Exhibit 5-1).

At the same time an instructor is determining this information, the instructor, course coordinator, and/or the training institute administration should also be setting the program's goals (see Chapter 11). These goals and objectives set the performance standards for the faculty of the training program. These are created when the lesson plan is being written. These performance objectives are designed to measure the quality of instruction during a training program. Chapter 11 provides specific details for establishing these objectives and offers a comprehensive program evaluation process. It is important to remember to establish these program objectives when the lesson plans are being written. Otherwise, the validity of the information that is attained can be questioned.

Having identified the type of students and their literacy levels, and having developed the goals for a program, the behavioral objectives are the next area to develop.

"The Blueprints": Behavioral Objectives

The blueprints for a house tell a contractor how to build the house. The behavioral objectives tell the instructor how to write the lesson plan, prepare the lesson materials, teach the material, and evaluate the learning

Exhibit 5-1

Student Reading Level and Lesson Material

Matching the lesson material to the reading level of the student is vital. An instructor can use various mechanisms to determine the reading level of the lesson material. A different set of mechanisms is used to determine the reading level of the students.

The Gunning-Fog Index, the Fry Method, and the Flesh Kincaid Scale are some of the diagnostic tools that an instructor can use to determine the reading level of a textbook or any other written course material. For most training programs, technical information should not exceed the 11th- or 12th-grade reading level.

Standardized prose literacy examinations can be used to determine a student's reading level. The lesson plan and course material can be designed to match the student's reading level. Matching the student's reading level to the course material improves the learning experience for the students.

experience. The importance of well-written behavioral objectives cannot be overstated. In almost every chapter of this book, behavioral objectives will be discussed. In each chapter, there is an explanation that will state how the behavioral objectives impact a particular topic. For example, Chapter 10 has an extensive explanation of the relationship between the behavioral objectives and the development of an examination. To avoid repeating information, this chapter will focus on the construction of the behavioral objectives. The use of objectives throughout the lesson plan will be highlighted.

Behavioral objectives for a lesson plan are created by the instructor or by the instructional team that will be teaching a particular lesson. To begin writing a set of behavioral objectives, identify a national, state, or locally developed teaching curriculum for the lesson that is being taught. Find the behavioral objectives and read them. An instructor should use each of a standardized curriculum's objectives. Using the U.S. DOT EMT-B National Standard Curriculum as an example, the EMT-B objectives are the minimum expectations that an instructor, training institute, or accrediting agency will expect students to meet. The key word here is *minimum*. If a training institute or accrediting agency desires a higher level of performance, the objectives can be rewritten to reflect this higher level of knowledge, performance, or understanding.

If instructors are writing a lesson plan that does not use a standardized curriculum, they must develop objectives based on their research of a topic. Research is vital when writing a lesson plan. Look in textbooks, reference manuals, and trade journals. Review the information and identify the areas of primary interest to the lesson's topic. After this research is completed the behavioral objectives can be written.

The purpose for writing a behavioral objective is to identify the student's behavior that is to be changed.[1] The only way an instructor can determine if a student has learned the information is to see a change in the student's behavior; in other words, it must be measurable. Writing an objective is based on the observation of this change in the student's behavior.[2] If a student cannot recognize when to use a wraparound short backboard, the goal is to change the student's behavior so that a student can recognize to use the device.

Using the wraparound short backboard example, the following is an example of a behavioral objective:

4
<u>At the conclusion of the spinal stabilization session</u>, students

1   2
will be able <u>to recognize situations in which the wraparound</u>

3
<u>short backboard is indicated 100 percent of the time.</u>

We will use this example to explain an objective's components. The four components are:

1. Action (behavior) verb
2. Content criteria
3. Condition (performance standard)
4. Audience

1. THE ACTION VERB

This verb states the behavior or activity that is to be learned by the student. The verb must be able to be measured; it must be able to be seen. The importance of the verb cannot be understated. The verb is the component that controls the type of learning that an instructor wants the students to accomplish.[3] If an instructor wants students to be able to recognize situations in which the wraparound short backboard is indicated, that is the level of learning that will be expected.

Action verbs are the product of one of three learning domains:

- Cognitive (knowledge)
- Psychomotor
- Affective

---

[1]U.S. Dept. of Transportation EMT Instructor Curriculum (Washington, D.C.: U.S. Government Printing, 1988).

[2]Ibid.

[3]Ibid.

It is the verb that controls what and how much is learned by a student. The verb determines the level of knowledge or ability that a student is requested to display.

Knowledge (Cognitive) Domain

The cognitive domain deals with behaviors that require mental or brain abilities. The taxonomy of educational objectives, illustrated in Figure 5-2, shows how students learn "knowledge."[4] The taxonomy can be viewed like an upside down pyramid. The most complex cognitive learning is located at the top of the pyramid. The taxonomy requires multiple pieces of information layered upon each other, which are learned from the starting point at the bottom of the pyramid, known as the knowledge or recall level.

Learning is based on these levels of understanding. Referred to as the cognitive domain, a student learns information from various levels of their understanding. The "knowledge" level (recall) is the simplest and the "evaluation" level (problem solving) is the most difficult level of understanding. The following description outlines each level of the taxonomy objectives:

- *Knowledge:* Ability to assemble all terms, facts, memorization of material, and recall of information necessary for other levels of learning. Example: "Identify the wraparound short backboard device."
- *Comprehension:* Ability to use knowledge and interpret, or translate the information. Example: "Recognize situations where the wraparound short backboard is indicated."
- *Application:* Ability to apply the information, to use the knowledge and comprehension, to apply the information to new situations. Example: "Demonstrate the application of the wraparound short backboard."

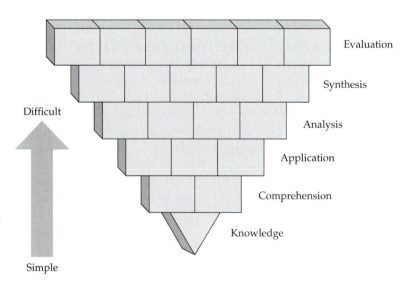

Figure 5-2
Bloom's Taxonomy of Educational Objectives.

---

[4]Benjamin S. Bloom, *Taxonomy of Educational Objectives,* bk. 1, *Cognitive Domain* (New York: Longman, 1956).

- *Analysis:* Ability to break down the information into components and look at each component and identify how it impacts the whole knowledge. Looking at elements and the relationships. Example: "Compare and contrast situations when a wraparound short backboard is or is not indicated."
- *Synthesis:* Ability to reassemble the information in a new manner. Abstract thinking and creativity are often used. Example: "Prepare a scenario that illustrates other uses of the wraparound short backboard device."
- *Evaluation:* Ability to make judgments, critiques, appraisals of the methods or procedures that are used. Example: "Following the completion of the scenario, evaluate the use of the wraparound short backboard device on an entrapped vehicle crash victim."

Exhibit 5-2 identifies verbs associated with each taxonomy level.[5] The taxonomy becomes the determinant for writing the entire lesson plan. If an instructor wants a student only to recall information, then the behavioral objective will contain an action verb associated with basic knowledge. However, if the instructor wishes students to be able to participate in problem-solving situations, then analysis, synthesis, and evaluation levels are to be used. Action verbs from these levels will be used to write the behavioral objectives to solve a problem situation.

The taxonomy of educational objectives provides an instructor with the ability to design the degree of learning that a student needs to solve a situation like the one described next. Objectives and teaching methods that stress minimum learning do not allow students to develop learning skills to solve real-life problems. Only when an instructor takes the time to develop behavioral objectives that stimulate students and encourage them to think for themselves will effective learning occur. This is the reason why so much emphasis is placed upon well written objectives—they are the lesson plan.

EXAMPLE

For example, Figure 5-3 illustrates an automobile accident. However, the auto has gone over a bridge and is submerged in water. If students are not challenged in the classroom to problem solve situations like these, then in real life their performance may be less successful and may be harmful to themselves and to others around them.

Psychomotor Domain

Psychomotor refers to the physical use of knowledge. There are basic components that an instructor must be aware of prior to a student performing a skill:

1. *Gross Body Movements:* The ability to move arms, shoulders, and legs in a coordinated manner, not to cause injury.

---

[5]Jerrold E. Kemp, *Instructional Design: A Plan for Unit and Course Development* (Belmont, Calif: Fearon/Janus/Quercus, 1977); FoxValley Technical College, its.foxvalley.tec.wi.us/iss/curric-assessment/column.html., 2000.

Exhibit 5-2

Taxonomy of Educational Objectives

ACTION VERBS

KNOWLEDGE

arrange	order	indicate	review
define	recognize	match	select
label	list	outline	state
name	recall	quote	trace
memorize	repeat	read	write

COMPREHENSION

classify	locate	add	express	select
discuss	describe	associate	summarize	indicate
identify	review	explain	visualize	translate

APPLICATION

apply	acquire	complete	discover	illustrate
operate	adapt	construct	examine	modify
choose	avoid	demonstrate	express	use
practice	change	determine	handle	prepare

ANALYSIS

analyze	differentiate	confirm	investigate
contrast	compare	ensure	prioritize
examine	experiment	explain	relate
criticize	diagram	group	select
question	calculate	infer	summarize

SYNTHESIS

assemble	organize	arrange	facilitate	portray
manage	construct	categorize	format	prescribe
create	prepare	cope	generalize	rearrange
design	formulate	develop	handle	revise
compose	set up	explain	modify	write

EVALUATION

appraise	assess	determine	predict	support
judge	compare	discriminate	rank	test
evaluate	conclude	interpret	rate	validate
score	counsel	measure	select	verify

Material discussed in the U.S. Department of Transportation EMT Instructor Curriculum, 1988, and from the Pennsylvania Department of Health EMT/Rescue Instructor Curriculum.

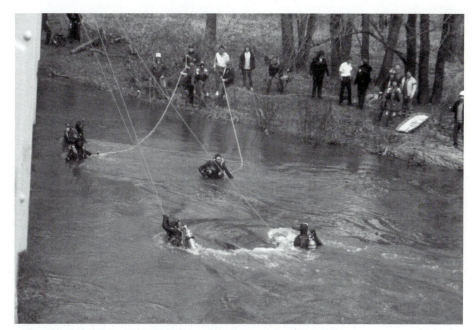

Figure 5-3
Ambulance 102, Rescue 5, respond to a vehicle accident at the bridge. The component left out is that the vehicle is in the water!

2. *Fine Movements:* Using hands, fingers, hand–eye coordination, and hearing to accomplish delicate procedures.
3. *Speech Behavior:* Using sound and body gestures to deliver a specific message or statement.
4. *Nonverbal Communication:* Facial expressions, gestures, and noncontrolled body movements.[6]

A student goes through different learning phases when learning a skill. The phases are:

1. *Imitation:* Observes the skill and attempts to repeat it.
2. *Manipulation:* Performs a skill based on instruction rather than observation.
3. *Precision:* Performs a single skill or task correctly.
4. *Articulation:* Combines multiple skills together.
5. *Naturalization:* Performs multiple skills correctly all the time.[7]

Before a skill objective can be written, an instructor should identify how a student should perform a skill. This is accomplished by using a task analysis. A task analysis identifies the steps involved in performing the skill.[8] For example, setting up/assembling the power hydraulic spreading

---

[6]William A. Mehrens and Irvin J. Lehmann, *Measurement and Evaluation in Education and Psychology,* 2nd ed. (New York: Holt, Rinehart and Winston, 1978).

[7]R. J. Armstrong, et al., *Developing and Writing Behavioral Objectives* (Tucson, Ariz., Educational Innovators Press, 1970).

[8]Mehrens and Lehmann, *Measurement and Evaluation in Education and Psychology.*

tool system, performing one-rescuer CPR, or connecting a fire hose to a hydrant and flowing water all would require a detailed description of the tasks needing to be completed in a specific sequence. Not all skills use a step-by-step approach. For complex skills an instructor might be interested in a comprehensive approach, rather than a step-by-step approach. The instructor must be familiar with the skills that will be performed and write the behavioral objectives corresponding to the task analysis. Also, do not forget about including any conditions or performance standards. The following example shows two different psychomotor objectives:

Comprehensive Skill Approach
The rescue captain will demonstrate an effective sizing up and identification of potential hazards throughout the simulated vehicle accident scenario, while coordinating personnel and equipment to effect the access, disentanglement, and safe extrication of the patients inside the vehicle.

Step-by-Step Skill Approach
Two rescue students will be given a complete air chisel system and air supply. The students will identify which student will operate the tool and which student will operate the air supply, followed by demonstrating the correct assembly sequence of the air chisel system beginning with:

1. Wear full protective clothing.
2. Connect the air regulator to the air supply.
3. Close the regulator valve and turn on the air supply and confirm the incoming pressure (in pounds per square inch [psi]).
4. Connect the high-pressure air chisel hose to the regulator and to the air chisel hammer.
5. Engage a chisel blade, suited for the type of metal to be cut, into the chisel hammer and manually assure the blade is engaged, constantly pointing the hammer at the ground.
6. Identify the type of metal and set the regulator gauge to the proper setting and open the regulator flow valve.
7. Cut the metal sufficiently to accomplish the intended objective.
8. Avoid prying with the chisel while cutting.
9. Disassemble the system by closing the air supply valve and relieving the pressure through the air hammer pressed against a hard object. Then disassemble in the reverse order used for assembly.

The skill behavioral objective is written in the same format as the knowledge objective. When writing a skill objective, the objective must be specific, so that all the components that are to be learned are identified. Additionally, any physical capabilities or other components necessary to perform the skill must be identified.

Some of the commonly used Action Verbs used in the psychomotor domain are:[9]

---

[9]FoxValley Technical College, its.foxvalley.tec.wi.us/iss/curric-assessment/column. html., 2000.

adjust	apply	assemble	break down	build	change
close	connect	construct	demonstrate	design	drill
follow	hook	load	locate	hammer	loosen
operate	pull	push	repair	replace	use

Affective Domain

The affective domain deals with attitudes, emotions, or values. The taxonomy of the affective domain identifies five levels of understanding.[10]

1. *Receiving:* Students are aware of something in their environment.
   Getting the students to pay attention.
2. *Responding:* Students display a behavior associated with an experience.
3. *Valuing:* Students show an active involvement or commitment.
4. *Organization:* Students accept a new value as theirs and set specific goals.
   Students compare and contrast their values to others'.
5. *Characterization by value:* Students act and use their new value.

A student's understanding or feelings about a lesson can be assessed by using the affective domain objectives.[11] The instructor must use keen observation skills to identify a student's reaction to a situation. Action verbs associated with the affective domain are:

accepts	participates	shares	judges
attempts	challenges	praises	volunteers

The following are examples of affective domain objectives:

- The student freely volunteers for extra credit projects.
- The student attempts to explain information without guidance from the instructor.
- The student accepts responsibility to act out the role of the crew chief during the scenario.
- The student participates in scheduled activities with vigor and energy.

When students learn information, they learn and react to information in multiple learning domains. The three domains have been separated to focus attention on the unique characteristics associated with each domain. In actual practice, an instructor might use all three domains to teach a basic concept.

---

[10]D. Krathwohl, B. Bloom, and B. Masia, *Taxonomy of Educational Objectives*, Handbook 2, *Affective Domain* (New York: David McKay, 1956).

[11]A. J. Harrow, *Taxonomy of the Psychomotor Domain* (New York: David McKay, 1972).

2. CONTENT REFERENCE

The second component of a behavioral objective is the content reference. Whenever an objective is being written, following the action verb will be a statement about the subject that is to be learned. In the example,

4
<u>At the conclusion of the spinal stabilization session</u>, students

1   2
will be able <u>to recognize situations in which the wraparound</u>

3
<u>short backboard is indicated 100 percent of the time.</u>

The content reference is "situations in which the wraparound short backboard is indicated." There will always be a verb and a content reference in an objective. The other two components may or may not be included in every behavioral objective, based upon the material that is being learned.

3. PERFORMANCE STANDARD

Whenever a student is being asked to perform a competency-based objective, this component becomes a requirement. The performance standard establishes the minimum performance criteria that will be accepted. In the example, the student is to attain a 100 percent recall of the information. It should be noted that whenever an objective is written, unless it is noted otherwise, it is assumed that the performance standard will be evaluated at 100 percent. Setting performance standards establishes a degree of competency assessment that an instructor can use to measure the degree of behavioral change. The variables usually associated with a performance standard component are time, accuracy, and quality of workmanship.[12]

4. CRITERIA OR CONDITIONS

This component, like the performance standard, may or may not be used in the behavioral objective, based on the material being presented. This component sets any additional requirements, information, or other details that help to clarify the behavioral objective for the students. Whenever it becomes necessary to provide specific information about the behavior, add the information as a criterion or condition for the behavioral objective.

Behavioral Objective Rules

Here are some rules to use when writing behavioral objectives.

Written First, Not Last   Sometimes a particular subject motivates an instructor. Often the behavioral objectives end up being written as an after-

---

[12]Mehrens and Lehmann, *Measurement and Evaluation in Education and Psychology.*

thought or not at all. No matter how powerful a subject may be, an instructor cannot forget the basics. The behavioral objectives form the foundation of the lesson plan. A house cannot be built without a foundation. Neither can a lesson plan be built without sound behavioral objectives. The behavioral objectives are written first, then the rest of the lesson plan and course materials are decided upon. A weak foundation equals a weak lesson plan.

Measurable Objectives   For an objective to be considered a behavioral objective, the objective must identify a specific behavior that can be observed. Knowledge and psychomotor objectives clearly meet this criterion. Affective objectives are not as easily observed and do not meet traditional definitions of a behavioral objective. By using rating scales and observational charts instructors can assess affective objectives.

Being measurable means that the objective consists of an action verb, identifies specific content criteria, often has a condition, and may state a performance standard. These components make the objective measurable.

SWBAT or LWBAT   When writing a behavioral objective, the objective is to be written in terms for the students. SWBAT stands for "student will be able to" and LWBAT means "learner will be able to." When writing a series of objectives, it is appropriate to begin the objectives with the SWBAT or LWBAT phrase. This condition states that a student is capable of accomplishing the stated objective.

An objective not written in student terms cannot be assessed by a student-oriented examination. To be considered a behavioral objective, the objective must be written in terms that reflect the student's behavioral change.[13]

Setting the Level of Understanding   An instructor determines the level of knowledge that students are expected to attain. This level becomes the overall difficulty level for the lesson. Objectives (specifically the action verb) set the learning level. A level that is set above the literacy level of the students can result in a poor learning experience. Objectives set too low will also result in a poor learning experience. The instructor must design the objectives to be challenging and obtainable.

Stating the Objectives   It is not important just for the instructor to know the behavioral objectives, but the students should be made aware of the behavioral objectives. At the beginning of each class, the instructor should outline the behavioral objectives that will be covered during the class session. This serves several purposes:

1. Students can track their understanding of the material.
2. Students can use the objectives to place emphasis upon studying habits for future examinations.

---

[13]U.S. Dept. of Transportation EMT Instructor Curriculum (Washington, D.C.: U.S. Government Printing, 1988).

3. Students will know how much material is left to cover.
4. The important aspects of the training program will be emphasized.

In addition to these purposes, behavioral objectives benefit the training institute and instructor in the following ways:

1. Instructors can track a student's learning development.
2. Instructors can track the classes' learning development.
3. The training institute can measure the instructor's effectiveness based upon the ability of the students to meet the objectives.
4. The overall program evaluation program can use the objectives to measure the effectiveness and efficiency of the program.

Lesson Plans

If the objectives are a building's blueprints and foundation, the lesson plan becomes the actual building. Built according to the behavioral objectives, the lesson plan identifies the creation and the conduct of the entire lesson. The lesson plan lists the objectives, provides a content outline, lists and describes AV aids, identifies the teaching methods, plus many more components that make a lesson plan.

Lesson Plan Components

A lesson plan assembles the lesson components into an organized format. Certain components tend to be commonly seen and expected in most lesson plans. Keep in mind that no one lesson plan is designed exactly the same. Instructors incorporate their personalities and style into their lesson presentations. The components of a lesson plan include:

Area 1: Title Section
- Title
- Lesson number
- Lesson date developed/revised
- Total time
- Instructor's name
- Course title
- Number of instructors required for the lesson

Area 2: Behavioral Objectives
- Knowledge objectives
- Skill (psychomotor) objectives
- Affective objectives

Area 3: Content Outline
- Organized listing of the presentation material

- Identification of any support material (AV aids, handouts, etc.) in the lesson
- Instructor notes (personal-style–oriented notes)
- Administrative notes (breaks, teaching methods, room setup, etc.)
- Oral questions and student evaluation
- Review of previously learned material from former lessons

Area 4: Support Materials
- AV materials and equipment needed for the lesson
- Classroom type and setup for the lesson
- Support equipment needed (medical, fire, or rescue training equipment)
- Administrative material (number of student exams, handouts, course evaluation forms, etc.)
- Reference materials used to write/supplement the lesson plan

Area 5: Additional Skill Lesson Components. Content outline that describes in detail the following elements:
- Steps of the skill
- Physical movements
- Cues for correct performance/errors
- Alternate methods
- Introduction of the skill
- Description of the practice (unsupervised/supervised)

AREA 1: TITLE SECTION

This portion introduces the lesson. The lesson's title, total time for the lesson, number of instructors needed for the lesson, and the lesson number, if it is one of several lesson plans being used throughout a course, are included in this section. The instructor who developed the lesson plan is listed, along with the date the lesson was initially developed. Also included is a listing of any revision dates. Updating the lesson plan on a regular basis provides the instructor who uses the lesson plan with an easy reference to the last revision date of the material.

AREA 2: BEHAVIORAL OBJECTIVES

This section identifies a lesson's behavioral objectives. Any knowledge, skill, or affective objectives are identified. This section is usually started using a phrase such as, "Students will be able to . . ." (SWBAT or LWBAT). This phrase reinforces who the objectives are written for, the students. The objectives should be listed separately. This separation reinforces the learning domains that are being taught during a lesson. The objectives determine the content and conduct of the lesson plan and should be listed at the beginning of the lesson plan.

AREA 3: CONTENT OUTLINE

This section is the "meat and potatoes" of the lesson plan. Most lesson plans are constructed using an outline format. An outline format lists the lesson material by its major topic, subtopics, topic information, and subtopic information. The following is an example of an outline:

   I. Lesson Plan
      A. Title section
         1. Title
         2. Lesson number
         3. Total lesson time
         4. Instructor's name
         5. Initial date/revision date
             a. Identify any revisions to the lesson plan
            b. Update the lesson plan to keep it current and up to date
            c. Behavioral objective
         6. S.W.B.A.T.
         7. Knowledge objectives
         8. Skill (psychomotor) objectives
         9. Affective objectives

Using the outline format instructors can quickly look at a topic area and identify the lesson material that they are covering. The outline should contain the essential lesson information needed to teach the lesson plan. An outline does not replace an instructor's lecture notes. Save specific details and personal notes for the lesson's lecture notes. The lesson plan should indicate those places where lecture notes are being used.

In addition to the content outline, there are other components that directly support the outlined material. Included is an introductory outline. The components from area 1—namely, lesson title and the time of the lesson—are identified. The behavioral objectives should be stated to the students, so that everyone knows what is going to be covered in the lesson. Previously learned materials should also be reviewed in the introductory outline. A final component is taking care of any administrative matters; that is, passing back assignments, organizing the classroom, taking attendance, and reviewing an examination. The introductory outline provides a starting point for the lesson plan.

Administrative, personal, and support material notes help an instructor identify the classroom setup, a specific method of instruction, when to break, a particular AV aid, and so on. These are nothing more than simple reminders for the instructor. This mechanism is used to keep the instructor on track with the lesson plan.

A final supplement to the content outline can be oral questions, or other student evaluation mechanisms. Often an instructor wants to stimulate a discussion by using a structured question. Some instructors include these discussion questions in the content outline at the point where they want to ask the question. Quiz reminders are also included as a portion of the outline. In most cases, these notes are nothing more than reminders for the instructor, but they keep the instructor and the presentation on track.

AREA 4: SUPPORT MATERIALS

This section could also be referred to as the logistics section. How much, how many, when, and where are the type of questions that find their answers in this section. Any support material (e.g., audiovisual equipment, audiovisual software, training equipment, facilities, classroom setup) is to be identified in this section. Often, instructors set this section up like a checklist. As they are preparing to teach the lesson, they review the equipment and supplies that will be needed for the lesson. This lessens the panic associated with forgetting a crucial piece of equipment for the lesson presentation.

An additional component of this section is a listing of the sources used to create the lesson plan. Often students ask where they can obtain additional information. Listing the lesson's resources also benefits the instructor when reviewing and updating the lesson plan.

These are just some of the elements to assist the instructor make a good lesson plan and presentation. The next section looks at the various lesson plan formats.

Lesson Plan Format

There is no one standard format for putting the information together. Insert the CD-ROM and click on "Lesson Plan Templates." Also on the CD-ROM is a "sample presentation." You will find examples of lesson plans and templates that can be used to start writing a lesson plan.

Paper size often acts as a determinant for an instructor. Lesson plans are usually written on $8\frac{1}{2} \times 11$-inch or $11 \times 8\frac{1}{2}$-inch paper. From that point on, it is up to an instructor to decide how to incorporate the elements of the lesson plan into the lesson plan format.

An instructor will often develop a personal preference for the placement of the lesson plan components, for example, whether to have, and/or when to have, instructor notes in the lesson plan. Each of the lesson plan components is decided on and placed into the lesson plan based on the instructor's needs.

The type of lesson plan format will be tailor-fitted to each instructor. Each of these examples incorporates the necessary lesson plan components, but is designed to fit the needs of the instructor. Whether it is sideways or up and down, as long as it contains the essential components, it will be a lesson plan.

A lesson plan is more than a teaching document. EMS personnel complete a patient care report as their written "legal" documentation of their patient encounter. For instructors, the lesson plan is an instructor's legal document to attest to what was and was not taught to students. Incorporated into the lesson plan should be a section that identifies when (date) and where the lesson plan was presented. Any updates or revisions to the lesson plan should be documented by a revision date and a summary of the revisions. Should the content of the lesson plan ever be questioned, this information will become invaluable to an instructor.

Lecture Notes

Lecture notes are the mechanism used to provide an instructor with specific detailed information during a presentation. A lesson plan is not intended to list every last detail. For specific referencing of material, instructors should use a set of lecture notes for this type of information.

Many instructors use 3 × 5-inch note cards. Specific quotes, questions, group discussions, AV aids, and the like are written out on these cards. An instructor can casually view the cards throughout a presentation, in the same manner that an instructor should view the lesson plan.

Both the lesson plan and lecture notes should be viewed as adjuncts to the lesson during a presentation. An instructor should not have to reference these adjuncts any more than is necessary. Frequent reading of lesson plan material or notes during a presentation is not considered to be a positive instructor characteristic. Instructors should use them for what they are intended, as reminders during a lesson presentation.

Training Curriculums

Depending upon the training institute, an instructor may be using lesson materials as a part of the institute's curriculums. What is a curriculum? In simple terms, a curriculum is a collection of lesson plans that are bound together to form a complete training program for a particular subject. Every school district, vocational school, or college has some type of curriculum. Instructors at these institutes use an established program of instruction, for example, American history, cosmetology, or an MBA program.

Emergency service instructors follow curriculums. EMS instructors primarily use the *U.S. Department of Transportation National Standard Curriculum* to teach first responder, EMT, and paramedic courses. Fire and rescue instructors use both national and state fire academy curriculums. Some states have modified their state training curriculums to exceed established national standards. Other states have designed their own curriculums for specific training programs.

As an instructor, seek out the training curriculum that is designed for your particular training program. Incorporate the objectives into your lesson plan; however, alter the objectives to meet your training institute's standard of performance. Often state/federal regulations do not permit a training institute to raise certain passing scores in state- and/or federal-regulated training programs. So it is advisable that you check with the state or federal agency responsible for the training program regulations to make sure your training criteria will comply with any specific regulations.

Some instructors find themselves with no previously created curriculum. They and the training institute staff must jointly decide on the teaching approach and then design the lesson plans and course materials for the new curriculums. This becomes a challenging process for an instructor who is fortunate to be a part of creating a new curriculum. As opposed to using someone else's ideas, the instructor's ideas and creativity can be used to construct the curriculum. It becomes a rare opportunity for most instructors. Any instructor who is provided the opportunity to develop a training curriculum should be encouraged to participate.

Summary

Whewwwww . . . and just how big is the house that was built? This chapter started out with an analogy: Building a house is like constructing a lesson plan. Building materials were substituted for educational concepts. Behavioral objectives, content research, and lesson plan development were the main materials used to design the lesson presentation.

Throughout the chapter, detailed information is provided for each component that is included in writing a lesson plan. The beginning of the lesson plan starts with well-written behavioral objectives. The entire lesson is dependent upon the objectives. From the initial instruction to the final examination, the objectives control the entire learning process.

The lesson plan format becomes a personalized format for each instructor. Examples and templates of lesson plan formats were identified.

For the art-oriented instructor, writing a lesson plan is a futile mission. However, for the science-oriented instructor, it is an essential aspect of the presentation. To have a balanced presentation, the instructor's "homework" assignment is to have adequately prepared lesson materials for the lesson presentation. If the art-based instructor can provide quality instruction with a one-page lesson plan while it takes the science-oriented instructor a five-page lesson plan to provide the same quality of instruction, these are differences that do occur in real-life settings. Lesson plans are the reflection of the instructor. Good instructors tend to have good lesson plans. A well-written lesson plan paves the way for quality instruction, which is the mission of any instructor.

How big is the house? The answer is, as big as you want it to be! It is an instructor's decision whether to build a "hunting cabin" or a "mansion." You, as the instructor, decide what the lesson plan will be. As a student, what are the wants or needs from a lesson presentation? An instructor is the architect of the lesson plan for the students. Although it is your decision as the instructor, design the lesson plan to fit the students. It is all a part of being a good instructor.

Chapter 6

Multimedia Systems and Educational Resources

➤ OBJECTIVES

- Identify and discuss the role of the instructor in becoming a user of multimedia systems.
  —Analyze how instructors select multimedia aids for a lesson.
  —Identify the attributes for using multimedia.
- Examine the equipment found in yesterday's, today's, and tomorrow's classrooms.
- Describe the operation of multimedia equipment.
- Identify various educational resources that are available.
- Describe how media can be a motivator for students.
- Compare and contrast the forms of media and identify their strengths and shortcomings.
- Identify the costs associated with the forms of media.
- Examine the influence that computer technology has had on the use of multimedia programming in the classroom.
  —Describe and discuss the use of PowerPoint-style programs with multimedia projection systems.
  —Identify the multimedia resources available through the Internet.

Motivation = learning. The first level (receiving) of the affective domain deals with gaining the attention of the student. Using multimedia systems programming allows instructors to gain and hold the student's attention. Do not forget the "art of the little things" when you want to hook 'em, the students, the first time! In previous chapters, it has been stated that when students become active participants in the learning experience they learn and retain more information than in passive learning situations. Through multimedia systems programming, students can learn and retain more information and have fun doing it. Using multimedia systems allows learning to come alive.

In our daily lives, media resources surround us. At home, work, in shopping malls, on the street corner, and in our classrooms, a variety of media resources are influencing our lives. Instructors must become technology savvy and provide students with learning situations that motivate and challenge their learning abilities. Using a comprehensive multimedia approach to instruction can aid instructors in motivating their students.

What is multimedia systems programming? How do instructors select the right multimedia aids for their students? Where do you find multimedia

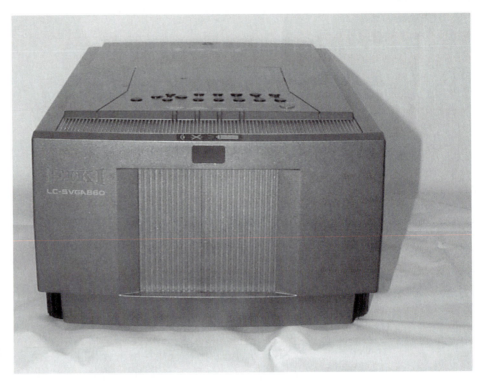

Figure 6-1
Multimedia system.

resources? And how are multimedia resources incorporated into the lesson plan? These questions will be answered in the next section (Figure 6-1).

Lesson Plan and Objectives

Regardless of the multimedia system or educational resource, it must meet the lesson plan's objectives. Multimedia programming and educational resources are identified only after the objectives have been written. Media aids are designed to support the lesson material, not to take its place. Too much is as bad as too little. An instructor must carefully plan the use of multimedia programming.

Planning the Educational Resources

Planning the educational resources is done when the lesson plan is being written. Selection of educational resources is based upon a series of determinants, such as

1. Behavioral objectives
2. Media effectiveness
3. Cost
4. Instructor's awareness of multimedia systems
5. Availability of the resources

Behavioral Objectives   Depending on the behavioral objective, the types of resources may be unlimited or limited. If an objective states, "Students

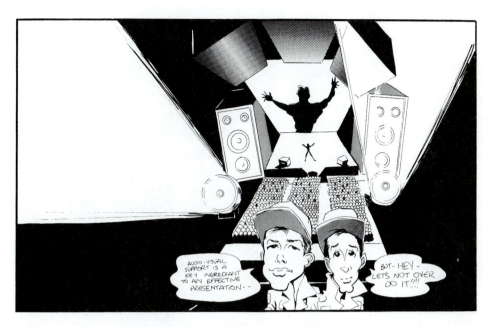

AV overkill. *Courtesy of the Baker Street Group.*

will evaluate the performance of Rescue Company A at the scene of an MVA," an instructor could use any of the following resources:

- Chalkboard drawing or overhead transparency of an accident scene
- Review of communication center audio tapes
- Still pictures or slides of the scene
- Actual videotape of the accident scene
- Computer simulation of an accident scene
- Field exercise with a simulated accident scene
- Ride-along program with a metropolitan based rescue service that allows students to actually evaluate the performance of Rescue Company A

This rescue lesson plan objective can be met by using any of the above resources. Meeting the objective is only one element to consider. The following media determinants must also be considered.

Effectiveness   The effectiveness of an educational resource is an important consideration. Examining the rescue objective, there is a varying level of student involvement, ranging from passive to interactive. Viewing overhead transparencies, slides, and listening to an audiotape are the least interactive methods. Viewing, discussing, and evaluating a videotape of an accident scene or using a computer accident simulation program would be more interactive, kind of middle-of-the-road. Participating as an observer at a rescue simulation or actual rescue scene would be the most effective. Note that all of the educational resources meet the rescue objective. The effectiveness of a media resource is measured in the amount of student involvement and a student's learning potential. For the rescue objective, educationally the most effective resources would be the rescue simulation or the actual ride-along program (Figure 6-2).

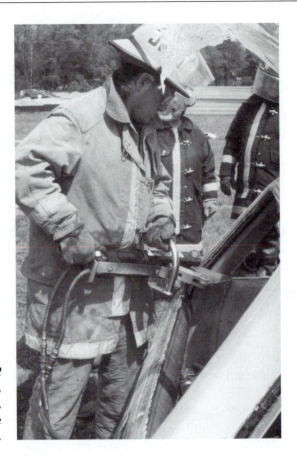

Figure 6-2
For learning to occur,
students need to see,
hear, touch, and use
equipment.

But what if there is not a metropolitan rescue department that can be used for a ride-along program? Or the instructor does not have access to a videotape of an accident scene? Although an educational resource may be effective, it may not be the most practical. Cost, availability of the resources, lesson-plan time constraints, and the instructor's familiarity with the educational resources can influence the effectiveness of a resource. Often an instructor must concede the level of effectiveness based on these factors.

Costs   There are costs associated with educational resources (Figure 6-3). Even though an audiovisual aid may be an effective resource, its cost may preclude its use. Let's look at some of the costs of different educational resources.

Training institutes provide instructors with access to a variety of educational resources. In a traditional classroom an instructor can expect to find a chalkboard or dry image board, projection screen, overhead projector, slide projector, TV/VCR, various training models, manikins, training equipment, maintenance/support equipment (e.g., power cords, spare bulbs), and instructional support resources (e.g., trade journals, reference books). Videotape or audiotape libraries are often available through the training institute. Each of these resources has a cost. When instructors use these resources, their costs are not usually considered. Actually, these instructional resources tend to be taken for granted. However, to a training institute, acquiring these aids has an instructional cost, one that is often large.

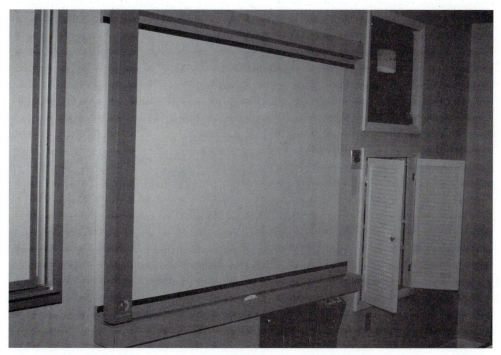

Figure 6-3
This electronic display board is a great instructional tool, but is found in few classrooms due to its expense.

The costs associated with the resources found in a traditional classroom could range from $25,000 to over $50,000 for each classroom. For advanced training programs, like paramedic courses, costs could be even more. In many of today's and tomorrow's classrooms, the traditional educational resources are supplemented with computer enhanced instructional aids, interactive computerized training manikins, and multimedia presentation systems. Computer labs/simulation rooms and multimedia rooms are being built by training institutes to meet the educational needs of the students. This means even more costs to a training institute.

Instructor Awareness   A training institute can have state-of-the-art educational resources, but if an instructor does not know how to use them their value is diminished. One of the purposes of this chapter is to introduce instructors to a variety of traditional and advanced educational resources. It is an instructor's responsibility to become aware of the educational resources that are available through the training institute. Instructors should familiarize themselves with the resources they will be using on a regular basis. Knowing what resources are available helps instructors to incorporate these resources into their lesson plans.

Availability   Just because a training institute has a particular educational resource does not necessarily mean that it will be available for an instructor's presentation. It might be used by another instructor or is no longer available. As soon as an instructor identifies an educational resource needed for the lesson plan, the resource should be acquired or reserved for the time period of the lesson. A few instructors have been known to have blundered by not checking the availability of an educational resource.

Time and Logistics   Instructors are often faced with limited time to cover a large number of behavioral objectives. The time is often complicated with logistical concerns. Using the rescue simulation as an example, the time and logistical coordination required to conduct a rescue simulation would be a time intensive activity. Thus, instructors need to make sure they have preparation time, classroom time, and logistical resources available to use any media resource.

Only after these determinants have been considered should an instructor decide upon an educational resource. Any one of these determinants can influence how instructors will present the material to their students.

Yesterday's, Today's, and Tomorrow's Resources

Many of the educational resources used in today's classroom will be called relics in tomorrow's classroom. Although a resource may still be physically usable, the educational appropriateness of the resource may make it unusable. For example, an instructor could use human anatomy flip charts to teach a human anatomy presentation. Or the instructor could use a computer animation program, like A.D.A.M. Essentials, and use the zoom feature to look at specific anatomical structures, pronounce medical terms, and show an animated 3-D image of the human anatomy. There will always be a new and improved gadget to replace an old standby educational resource.

Which educational media resources are already considered relics? Exhibit 6-1 identifies educational resources that are considered outdated and/or may have limited usefulness in today's classrooms. Exhibit 6-2 identifies educational resources that are not yet relics but could be added to the relic list. These "endangered resources" still have a use in the traditional classrooms, but could easily be replaced by a new gadget. Exhibit 6-3 lists some resources that are considered state-of-the-art. Today's and tomorrow's instructors need to keep aware of new educational resources. Every year brings new resources to learn about and use in educational institutes.

Using Multimedia Systems

When a lesson plan is being developed, an instructor identifies the educational resources that will be used to teach a lesson. Many of these resources (videotapes, slide-audiotapes, PowerPoint presentations, computer simulations) use both audio and visual mediums. These presentations can increase a learner's retention because they are multisensory in their design.

A multimedia presentation uses multisensory sources to present the lesson's material. Using a variety of media resources creates a multimedia presentation. The use of a storyboard is helpful when designing a multimedia presentation (Exhibit 6-4). A storyboard identifies the audio, visual, and written material used in a presentation. Storyboards can help an instructor effectively design multimedia presentations.

Exhibit 6-1

Relic Educational Resources	
RELIC EDUCATIONAL RESOURCES	**LIMITED USE**
16 mm film projector	Most films contain dated material.
35 mm filmstrip projector	Do not exist for most programs. Dated material.
Opaque projector	Useful for copying images onto a dry image board.
8-track tape player	Tapes do not exist.
Vinyl record player	Records do not exist.
8 mm movie camera	No usefulness.
Flip charts (anatomy charts)	Can be used in small group activities. Better resources exist.
Blackboards	Still used. Dry image boards are replacing blackboards. Advantages include no chalk dust and vivid color pens.
35 mm camera	Still used but rapidly being replaced with digital cameras.

Instructors must become familiar with the media resources that are available through their training institute (Figure 6-4). This section identifies a variety of media resources and explains how to use them before, during, and after a presentation. Insert the CD-ROM and click on the media resources button. Click on a media resource and you will see how to use the resource. Resources covered include:

- Slide projector
- Overhead projector and overlays
- TV/VCR/DVD
- Dry image board
- Projection screen
- Multimedia projector
- Digital camera
- Support equipment

Exhibit 6-2

Endangered Educational Resources	
ENDANGERED EDUCATIONAL RESOURCES	**TIMELINESS OF THE RESOURCE**
Cassette audio tapes	Still exist. CD-ROMs and other forms of digital audio devices provide better sound and recording quality.
TV sets and TV cable	Standard color TV sets are being replaced with digital TV, large screen TV, multimedia projectors, or flat screen TVs. The newer TVs augment the digital TV cable and digital satellite TV systems. The images are clear and crisp and the audio quality is awesome.
VCRs	Still exist. DVD systems provide crisp digital audio and video images. There is a growing compatibility between DVD players and computer technologies.
Slide projectors	Still exist. The use of multimedia projectors connected to computers that use PowerPoint type presentations is rapidly replacing 35 mm slides.
Overhead projectors	Still exist. Advanced computer/software and color printers allow instructors to design and use professional quality transparencies. Multimedia projectors, connected to a computer, can present the same images without using transparencies.

Exhibit 6-2 (cont'd.)

Endangered Educational Resources	
ENDANGERED EDUCATIONAL RESOURCES	**TIMELINESS OF THE RESOURCE**
Dry image boards	Still exist. Electronic image writing boards are replacing dry image boards because they can capture a written image before the image is erased.
Full body CPR manikins	Traditional full body CPR manikins have been replaced with torso models that are a fraction of the cost. An improved line of CPR manikins that use computers and DVD technology creates an almost living manikin.
½-inch VCR camera	Some exist but most have been replaced with 8 mm or digital video cameras.
Written textbooks/ reference materials	Emerging technologies such as e-books, e-ink, and the Internet are replacing many forms of printed material and may place them onto an endangered resource list.

Using Specialty Educational Resources

There are specialty educational resources that today's and tomorrow's instructors need to be acquainted with. These resources may not be available in every training institute. These resources reviewed are:

- Electronic Image Writing Board
- Satellite TV
- Internet Con-Ed and CD-ROM programming
- PowerPoint type presentations

Exhibit 6-3

State-of-the-Art Educational Resources

STATE-OF-THE-ART EDUCATIONAL RESOURCES	ADVANTAGES AND COMMENTS
Computers and software	Growing. More and more institutes are including lab sessions. New software programs are being developed to assist students and instructors.
Internet	Exploding. Invaluable resource for anyone associated with education, training, public safety, or emergency services.
Digital TV/flat screen TV	Replacing conventional TV sets. Sharp and crisp images and audio quality.
Multimedia projectors and PowerPoint type presentation software	Replacing traditional forms of media resources. Permits multiple sources of media to be used. Versatile software that allows instructors to design the media to fit their lesson plan material.
DVD and digital audio systems	DVD discs can be used on either computers or TV systems. CD-ROM recorders enable CDs to be burned and allow instructors to make their own audio and digital CDs.
Whiteboards and electronic image boards	Whiteboards and electronic image boards convert written images into a digital or written text. Whiteboards can be connected to Internet and video sources.
Digital still and video cameras	Digital images can be created instantly and incorporated into multimedia presentations or posted onto the Internet.

Exhibit 6-3 (cont'd.)

State-of-the-Art Educational Resources

STATE-OF-THE-ART EDUCATIONAL RESOURCES	ADVANTAGES AND COMMENTS
Digital flatbed scanner	Take any photo or written text, scan it, and turn it into a digital image.
Education and Con-Ed online or via CD	A four-walled classroom does not have to be used to take some training courses. More and more training courses are available via the Internet or on CD-ROM.
Satellite or Internet	Satellite and Internet courses are already available to many emergency service providers. Some provide two-way visual and audio feeds to make them an interactive learning experience.
Virtual reality programs	These computer simulations use graphics, sounds, and animations to create realistic environments. Virtual reality systems combine body sensors and a helmet-like viewer to allow the wearer to experience and interact with the computer.
E-ink and e-Books	Both are emerging technologies and can reform how students and instructors use printed media products. Instead of purchasing a hardback textbook, call up a textbook title on the Internet and download it into either product. See Chapter 12 for more information about both technologies.

Exhibit 6-4

Storyboard Example

Presentation Name: _____

Date Developed: ____/____/____

Presentation For: _____

Revision Date: ____/____/____

Resources Required:

____ Computer   ____ Multimedia Projector

____ PowerPoint Software   ____ Internet Access

____ Projection Screen   ____ External Speakers

AUDIO	VIDEO	SCRIPT	COMMENTS
(None)	PowerPoint Standard Background Blue Color Yellow Font Color	"Focus"	Presentation will review the use of PowerPoint software and how to use Internet hyperlinks.
(.wav audio of applause)	Fade in and have text slide from left. Clip art of computer and computer screen.	"Welcome to PowerPoint and Internet Hyperlinks"	
(None)	Dissolve. Program hyperlink to www.brady books.com.	"Brady Books" logo	Hyperlink demonstration. Connect to Internet prior to presentation.
(None)	Navigate through Pearson-Brady Internet site.	Show homepage and special features of the Pearson-Brady site.	

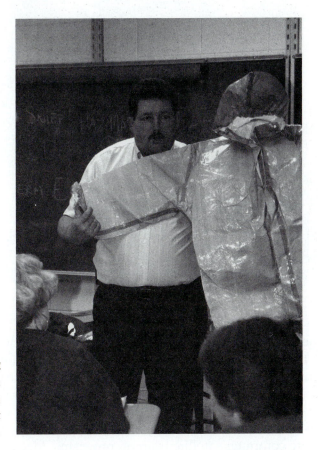

Figure 6-4
An instructor's demonstration uses a piece of equipment as a media resource.

ELECTRONIC IMAGE WRITING BOARD

Many an instructor has said, "Gee, I wish I could save the material that I have put onto the chalkboard." Well, someone took this saying to heart and invented the electronic image writing board.

The board surface looks like a normal dry image writing board, except that a large tube is mounted vertically on a track along the top and bottom of the board, and a printing panel is located at the bottom of the board. The instructor uses dry image pens to place the material onto the board. At the conclusion of the lesson presentation, instead of immediately erasing the material, the instructor depresses a button and the cylinder moves across the board. The printer then displays the image that was written on the board. The series of photographs in Figures 6-5, 6-6, and 6-7 shows an instructor putting information onto the board and then printing the information that was written on the board.

The electronic image writing board is not a piece of inexpensive equipment. A training institute and its instructors need to assess the benefits of having this board. From an instructor's viewpoint it is a dream come true. From a program administrator's perspective, it is a monetary issue. It can obviously solve the instructor's dilemma of losing material that is written

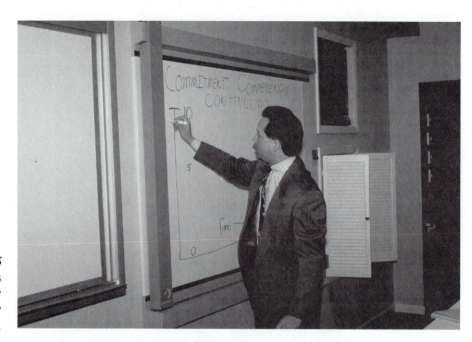

Figure 6-5
Instead of losing his
graph, this instructor
can save it for
later use.

on the board. The instructor can take the printed copy and make copies of it for the students. The board enhances the information exchange between the instructor and the students. It is obviously a great enhancement to a classroom. The cost of the unit may prohibit many training institutes from acquiring the unit. An analysis of how and where it will be used is useful in the assessment of the board. It is a new technology that is already being tied into computer satellite training programs. Many instructors may find

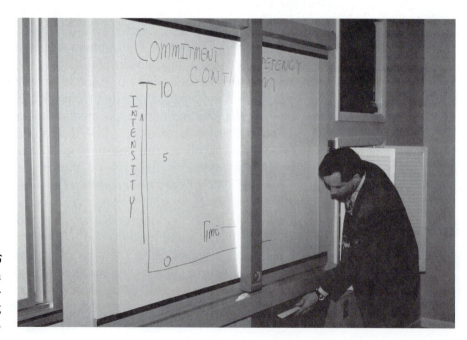

Figure 6-6
The scanner has been
activated and the in-
formation is being
prepared for printing.

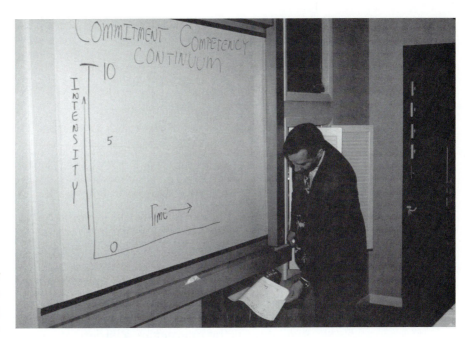

Figure 6-7
The image on the board is being printed out.

these boards in their classrooms as time passes. It may be the device to make the chalkboard obsolete.

SATELLITE TV

Limited only by the number of satellite receiving locations, an instructor can educate numerous students simultaneously in multiple worldwide locations. Linking multiple classrooms together at the same time, students learn material jointly, even if they are hundreds of miles away from each other. An expensive venture for a single training institute, satellite learning (also referred to as distance learning) can be a way to present the same lesson material to multiple students at the same time. Satellite programming is an option worthy of consideration. Universities, school districts, hospitals, and state agencies offer satellite programming. Sharing the costs between several training institutes can make this programming an affordable venture.

Enhanced systems allow the instructor and students to communicate audibly and visually. Additional enhancements include linking a whiteboard to the system so the classrooms can collectively share the same written information.

There are numerous methods for conducting a satellite program. Frequently used in satellite sessions, a "keynote presenter" delivers the main lesson material. At each satellite receiving location are local level instructors to review and expand upon the keynote presenter's material. An adaptation could be to have the main presentation outline how to perform a particular skill and then have local instructors actually conduct hands-on skill sessions.

Logistics associated with satellite-based education often limit its use. Broadcast and receiving equipment is expensive. Satellite time is often limited. There are studio and video production costs. Carefully planned and used, satellite programming can be an invaluable educational resource.

INTERNET CON-ED AND CD-ROM PROGRAMMING

In Chapter 12, the history and use of the Internet is discussed in detail. An emerging aspect available via the Internet or on CD-ROM is a variety of educational resources for initial or continuing education. Everyday there are interactive programs being developed that are changing how educators present information to their students.

The Internet is being used for initial and continuing education programming. Universities are offering classes, once offered on campus, online. Students located hundreds, even thousands, of miles away from a university can take college credit courses. Emergency service training programs are being developed for the Internet. For a fee, an emergency service practitioner can take an online continuing education course. An online test is taken, graded, and upon successful completion of the test, a certificate of completion is mailed to the practitioner.

Available via the Internet are a variety of educational resources related to emergency services. Using an Internet search engine, these resources can easily be identified. Fire, rescue, and EMS instructors can find just about anything. Photos, news stories, curriculum changes, instructional tips, games, crossword puzzles, simulations, plus many other resources can be found on the net.

At the Pearson-Brady Internet site, www.bradybooks.com, there are a variety of educational resources for students and instructors. One of the resources is interactive case study simulations, where EMS personnel react to realistic situations, based on their level of training. There are additional educational resources available at the site including CD-ROM programs.

There are a variety of computer CD-ROM programs available for use in emergency service programs. CD-ROM programs are multimedia-based programs. There are programs that are computer animations, others use digital video and audio clips, while others are more like a game or simulation. Instructors should review trade journals and online resources to keep updated on the latest programs that are available. Multimedia programs keep a student's interest and make learning fun.

POWERPOINT TYPE PRESENTATIONS

If you want to grab and keep your students' attention, design and use a multimedia software program like Microsoft's PowerPoint. PowerPoint presentations can be developed around an instructor's lesson plan. A presentation can be a "slide" type of presentation or can be a multimedia resource presentation. PowerPoint can be used as a self-tutorial computer program or can be used to coordinate multiple multimedia presentations.

Insert the CD-ROM and click on the tutorial program ("Learning PowerPoint with Vern"), which is created with PowerPoint. The program shows some of the uses of PowerPoint presentations.

PowerPoint contains a development wizard that is used to create basic "slide" programs. Using a multimedia projector, an instructor advances

PowerPoint images by using the projector's remote control (insert the CD-ROM, click on "Media Resources"). An animation feature allows an instructor to choose how each slide and text is transitioned. Additional features control whether the text is lit or dimmed, appears automatically or only when the remote is clicked.

Foreground and background colors of each slide can be selected. Pre-developed templates can be used to select the type of information that is being presented. These include the title, subtitle, bulleted lists, clip art with bullets, animated charts, and even digital movies. Instructors can use the predesigned templates and backgrounds or they can design their own templates and slide transition effects.

The true power of PowerPoint is its diversity to integrate multiple forms of media into a single presentation format. Sounds, digital images, movies, charts, diagrams, and even links to Internet sites can be incorporated into a PowerPoint presentation. An instructor has unlimited resources that can be accessed during a lesson presentation. Identify an instructional issue and it can be incorporated into a PowerPoint presentation. (Insert the CD-ROM and click on the "Power of PowerPoint".)

A PowerPoint presentation can be placed onto an instructor's laptop computer, floppy discs, CD-ROM, or sent to the Internet. It can be used as a self-tutorial computer interactive program. The uses of PowerPoint are endless.

PowerPoint is a tremendous asset, if used correctly. How a PowerPoint presentation is ultimately used is identified in an instructor's lesson plan. Whether it is a PowerPoint presentation, any media resource, or educational resource, it must complement, not replace, an instructor's lesson plan. As useful as a resource can be, if it is not used correctly it can end up being useless.

Summary

While the use of various media resources enhances training programs, the instructor must select those forms of media that will meet the lesson objectives, will be effective in delivering the message, and will be available for the presentation.

Different types of media resources were identified and discussed in detail. Each of the media resources has positive and negative aspects. Each one operates slightly differently from another. Some need extensive preparation to use, others can be easily set up and used.

Media and educational resources are used to stimulate and motivate students. Media can deliver a message in a way unlike any other technique. An instructor who can select and use media and educational resources effectively is likely to have a classroom of motivated and educated students.

Reference Material

Pennsylvania Department of Health Rescue Instructor Curriculum (Harrisburg: The Department, 1983).

Chapter 7

Facility and Classroom Setup

➤ OBJECTIVES

- Identify how an instructor can create the mood for a presentation through the physical classroom surroundings.
- Identify the environmental factors that influence the effectiveness of a facility.
- Examine classroom setup styles.
- Identify instructional resources contained within a classroom.
- Identify logistics associated with the use of a classroom, indoor and outdoors.
- Compare traditional classrooms to a no-wall educational environment.

What makes a good learning environment? Answers:

1. Whether inside or outside, the environment needs to be free from distractions that adversely affect a student's ability to concentrate on the lesson material.
2. It must provide a feeling of safety for the students.

This chapter looks at how an instructor uses classroom environments to create positive learning experiences. We will also provide insight into what tomorrow's classroom may look like.

The Traditional Four-Wall Classroom

The traditional classroom paradigm is a course taught in a well-lit classroom; the room temperature is set to a comfortable level; there is easy access to rest rooms; and instructors have access to a variety of media, educational resources, and training supplies (Figure 7-1). Instructors set up their classroom based on the needs of their lesson plan. This section looks at factors that influence the traditional classroom.

ENVIRONMENTAL CONDITIONS

As long as instructors do not permanently redecorate the room, they can move items (not bolted to the floor) around to create the type of setting that is needed for their presentation. There are environmental factors that

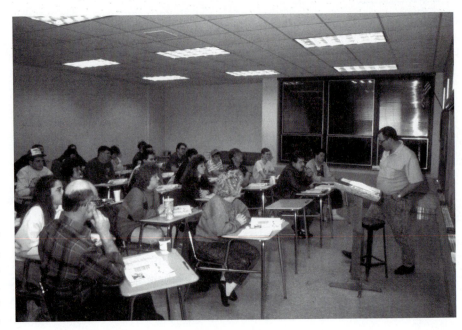

Figure 7-1
This is a view of a traditional classroom setup. Students are seated in rows of chairs that face the instructor. This setup is primarily used for lecture-style presentations.

an instructor can and cannot control within the classroom environment. These include:

1. Temperature
2. Distractions
3. Room safety
4. Lighting
5. Smoking
6. Access to rest rooms and break areas
7. Access to disabled students

Temperature

An instructor should try to make the classroom a comfortable temperature. Opening windows, closing doors, adjusting the heat/air conditioning thermostat, or turning the fan on/off are immediate ways an instructor can affect the climate of the room (Exhibit 7-1).

Exhibit 7-1

Cold Is Best!
Several studies conducted in the 1970s found that students who take written examinations performed better in rooms that were cool versus rooms that were too hot. The ideal room temperature for taking a test should be between 66 and 68 degrees Fahrenheit. Temperatures below or above tend to influence the student's ability to concentrate.

Instructors need to gauge the room temperature, not by how hot or cold they feel it is, but by how the majority of the students feel the temperature is within the room. Why not trust the instructor's judgment? Often, because instructors are walking and talking in the classroom, they may feel the room is comfortable when the rest of the class is shivering.

A room that is too hot is hard to cool, especially if the outside temperature is as hot as the inside temperature. Opening doors and windows will offer little help. If air conditioning is not available, an instructor can try a fan. However, the instructor will have to speak over the fan's noise, and this can end up being a bigger distraction. Both the instructor and students are affected by severe heat. An option is to move the session to an area that is cooler, even if it means moving the class outdoors under a shade tree.

If a building is perennially too cold or too warm, the instructor should bring this to the attention of the training institute. When the temperature, on a consistent basis, is adversely affecting students, the instructor will hear about it. Perhaps maintenance personnel can adjust the room's temperature, or the class can be moved to a different room free of the climate problem.

Distractions

An instructor can control some distractions, while others must be tolerated. An instructor cannot stop a freight train's whistle and noise from interrupting the class. But an instructor might try moving to a different room if it is a significant distraction. Another option may be to take breaks according to train schedules.

Anything that interferes with a lesson presentation is considered a distraction. Commonly seen distractions within emergency service training programs include students wearing alerting pagers, radios, and phones, the fire siren sitting atop the classroom, students or personnel walking in the hallway, excessive talking in class, and noise outside the classroom. Any of these factors can cause a distraction to the lesson presentation.

Room Safety

Educational environments must be safe. Student and instructor safety is more important than any educational component of a lesson; yes, even more important than the behavioral objectives!

Traditional classrooms, for the most part, are safe learning environments. A classroom facility must meet local safety codes and be free of any known structural problems, such as weak flooring or leaky ceilings. Classrooms with structural problems should not be used, based on the potential safety concerns.

Effective learning cannot occur when a presentation is being conducted in an unsafe classroom environment. Safety is the number one concern of a training program; everything else becomes secondary.

Lighting

How is the lighting in your classroom? Are the lights fluorescent or incandescent? Where are the light switches located? Are any lights burned out? Are they flickering? This section looks at how the lighting in a classroom can be a distraction, or at least an inconvenience, to an instructor and the students, and it examines the use of alternative lighting for specialty presentations.

The room should be lit well enough for the students to easily see the material. If a room is too dark, except when AV equipment is being used, the darkness becomes a distraction for many students. Some students may have difficulty seeing material in dark environments and a poorly lit classroom will only worsen their difficulty. The instructor should turn on the lights and see how well lit the room is upon first entering the room. If lights are burned out, contact the training institute maintenance personnel.

In a theatrical production, the role lighting plays is crucial. Lighting is used to set the mood of a scene and creates the desired effects for a production. Instructors, too, need to realize the impact that lighting has on their educational atmosphere and how they can create the mood for a lesson presentation. Just like in a theatrical setting, an instructor can use lighting to influence the lesson presentation. When an instructor is using AV equipment, like a slide projector, the lights must be turned off. But if lights are on different light switches one set of lights can often be left on. The room does not have to be totally darkened and the instructor can maintain eye contact with the students. If a classroom has variable incandescent lights, the lights can be dimmed for AV aids, as in a movie theater, and the students will still be able to see within the classroom (Exhibit 7-2). Fluorescent lights, at full strength, are needed when students are involved in activities that require precise vision. Activities such as taking written examinations, learning a skill, or presenting a tabletop demonstration require full-strength lighting. If a special lighting intensity is being used to set the mood for a lesson presentation it should be included in the lesson plan.

Smoking

Most training institutes do not permit smoking inside the building or allow it only in specifically designated rooms. In any case, during an actual class session, there should be a no smoking policy. It is extremely annoying to those who do not smoke, and it creates an unnecessary distraction. Students or instructors who smoke should do so during breaks in designated smoking areas.

Exhibit 7-2

An Economy Approach to Mood Lighting

If a training site only has on–off lights that cannot be controlled by a variable controller, here's an idea for being able to set the "mood" in a classroom.

Get several "work lights" with semicircle reflectors. Attach a clip onto the light assembly. Place the lights onto chairs next to a painted wall. Shine the lights upward and toward the wall. This provides a soft lighting, especially useful when using AV aids.

Access to Rest Rooms and Break Areas

Whether it is an indoor or outdoor classroom, an instructor must assure that students have access to rest room facilities. If this means renting portable facilities for outdoor training sessions, this is an environmental factor that cannot be ignored. Regular break sessions, usually one every 1 to 1–1/2 hours, should be scheduled. This allows students time to go to the rest room and relax in the break area.

A break area, with refreshments, provides the students and the instructor with an "unwinding area." Many training institutes have access to vending machines. For those that do not, the instructor may suggest that the class bring in a coffee maker and establish a coffee fund.

Access to Disabled Students

A training facility, according to the federal Americans with Disabilities Act (ADA), must be accessible to handicapped students. Depending upon the type of training program, for example, a dispatcher-training program, an instructor's classes may include physically handicapped students. An instructor needs to offer assistance to the handicapped student as is warranted. Specific requirements regarding making assistance and accommodations available to handicapped students is addressed in the Americans with Disabilities Act.

Outdoor Training Facilities

For many emergency service courses, training programs do not use a traditional classroom. Instead, specialty training facilities, like burn buildings, rappelling towers, auto salvage yards, and other outdoor settings are frequently used. Even though a four-walled classroom is not being used, there are environmental and educational factors that need to be considered.

Let's review some of the educational, logistical, and environmental aspects.

1. Temperature
2. Distractions
3. Safety and safety officer
4. Lighting
5. Smoking
6. Access to rest rooms and break areas
7. Fluid replenishment
8. Environmental concerns
9. Transportation

TEMPERATURE

Instructors cannot control the outdoor temperature, but they can influence how students adapt to the outdoor conditions. When an environment is too hot or cold it can adversely affect a lesson presentation. There are actions that can be taken to lessen the affects in these environments.

For hot environments, aspects to consider include

- Shaded areas (trees, tents, etc.) for briefings and review sessions
- Access to drinking water, ice, and cooling towels
- Cooling machines, water hoses, or spray bottles
- Sunscreen and block for all students and instructors
- Appropriate dress for students and instructors
- Access to an air-conditioned building or apparatus

For cold environments, consider

- Appropriate layered dress for students and instructors
- Protected area for briefings and review sessions
- Warming areas (burn barrels, heaters)
- Access to water and appropriate fluids
- Access to a heated building or apparatus

An instructor should be prepared to react to changing environmental situations. Because a session starts out with tolerable conditions does not mean that the conditions will not change; they likely will, and usually not for the better. In these cases the instructor must be ready to implement measures to ensure the safety of students and fellow instructors.

DISTRACTIONS

Traffic noise, horns beeping, train whistles blowing, people talking and walking near training facilities, environmental conditions, plus many other noises or conditions can be distractions to an outdoor lesson presentation. Most of these distractions are not within the control of the instructor. Instructors must adapt their presentations to the distractions when conducting outdoor activities.

SAFETY AND THE SAFETY OFFICER

An instructor must pay close attention to the safety of everyone participating in the lesson presentation. Additional attention is warranted for field evolutions where live fires, rappelling, or the extrication of live victims from wrecked vehicles are being performed. This is not to say that accidents cannot occur in a controlled setting; they can and they do.

An account of one training institute's experience during a practical session attests to the need for classroom safety. The session was held at a traditional two-story fire station; the type of fire station with a brass firefighters' pole. A breakout station was placed in the room with the fire pole. During the session, a student fell down through the pole hole into the truck room. The student received only minor injuries, despite the potential for serious injury. Foresight may have prevented this accident by not having the breakout station in the pole room.

Satellite training facilities and resources need to be inspected for their safety. Vehicle gas tanks being removed, floors being reinforced and emergency exits being created in burn structures, and water supply sources being identified are some examples of the type of pre-presentation safety inspections that need to be performed.

Potential accidents and injuries that can be seen in emergency service training programs include

1. *Back injury:* Lifting patients or equipment beyond the individual's capability.
2. *Cuts/lacerations:* Broken glass, sharp metal, uncovered sharps, unprotected knife or ax blades, and so on.
3. *Eye/skin injuries:* Gasoline, hydraulic fluid, battery acid, hazardous materials, and so on, spilled on gloves, clothing, and then wiped onto the skin or into the eyes.
4. *Soft tissue injuries:* Falling through floors, falling off ladders, or being hit by falling debris.
5. *Contamination:* Unsterile needle sticks, unclean manikins, or unsterile IV fluids.

Potential accidents can be reduced by mandating and enforcing appropriate protective clothing and equipment (e.g., SCBA, bunker gear, sharps containers, and examination gloves) and safety standards. Assistant instructors need to be used to assure students receive appropriate and safe training.

An invaluable individual for field activities is a safety officer. This is a third party, divorced from the session, whose sole task is to observe, identify, control, and alleviate any safety hazards, even if it means stopping the session. With an extensive knowledge in the type of evolutions being performed, the safety officer is to have total control. The presence of this individual adds an extra level of safety to the session.

A third-party safety team should be used for especially hazardous activities. Live burns, simulated vehicle accidents, high-angle rescues, or confined-space rescues require the presence of veteran emergency personnel. Should something happen during a training session, they are there to assist. These personnel must have the use of separate emergency resources (water supply, rescue equipment, rescue lines). Because students are learning how to use the equipment or to follow specific procedures, failures often occur. The safety team is there to protect the students and instructors.

LIGHTING

Vehicle accidents, fires, and rescues do not happen only in well-lit areas. When outdoor training facilities are being used, supplemental lighting must be considered. If late day sessions are likely to extend into evening hours, lighting of the training areas will be necessary. Generators, lights, and cords will be required. These resources would be in addition to lighting available on rescue apparatus.

The entire training ground needs to be lit. Lighting helps improve safety and prevent lost equipment, and it can be used to create specific realistic settings. Conversely, there are some situations when instructors do not want the environment lit. Smokehouse environments are, of course, supposed to be dark. The smokehouse building is to be free from any light sources. The darker a smokehouse is, with the addition of sufficient quantities of heat and smoke, the more realistic a practice situation becomes for the student.

SMOKING

Specific smoking areas should be established. No smoking should be permitted during training sessions. Only in designated areas should smoking be permitted. In many field sessions there are hazardous materials present (gas, oils, kerosene). Great care must be used to limit the exposure of these materials to a fire source. With the potential safety concerns associated with emergency service training programs, smoking during a practice session is an unwarranted hazard.

REST ROOMS AND BREAK AREAS

Outdoor training facilities often do not have immediate access to rest rooms. When access to permanent rest room facilities is not possible, portable rest room facilities should be considered.

Where's lunch? What's for lunch? Provisions for breaks and refreshments are part of the logistics when using an outdoor training facility. Depending on the number of students and faculty, lunch can be a problem. Box lunches, sandwiches, salads, and similar items are good alternatives. Few fast food restaurants exist in remote and rural areas where many classes are held.

FLUID REPLENISHMENT

In very hot or even in cold environments, it is important that both the students and faculty drink plenty of fluids. Good old water works well. If available, a salt-replenishing fluid can be drunk. Cool shady areas should be selected and a break area established. Conversely, in cold temperatures, the break area should be sheltered and, it is hoped, heated. Even in cool temperatures, students in "bunker gear" sweat enough to cause a fluid deficit. A fluid replenishment solution should be drunk instead of a hot drink like coffee. An instructor needs to anticipate the climate for the program and prepare enough refreshments for both the students and faculty.

ENVIRONMENTAL CONCERNS

The concern here is not so much with the climate as with other outdoor factors. Depending on the type of training activity, the following environmental factors should be considered:

- Extremely dry conditions
- Unstable rock formations

- Unstable ground or loose soil
- High wind conditions
- Poisonous plants, insects, and animals
- High water or fast moving water
- Unstable ice or snow
- Poor weather conditions

Any of these factors can influence a training activity. Everyone involved with the training activity should be made aware of potential hazards (e.g., poisonous plants, rock formations).

TRANSPORTATION

Getting from Point A to Point B can be a challenge. Is there sufficient parking at the outdoor training site? Who can drive students and faculty to and from the site? Are a bus and other transportation vehicles needed? These and other transportation issues require answers before an instructor conducts the outside activity.

Room Setup

The classroom needs to be set up to fit the lesson presentation. For practical skill sessions, the tables and chairs need to be pushed off to the side. Special breakout rooms can be set up for skill sessions. A burn building needs to be inspected and any burning supplies assembled. The diagrams in Figure 7-2 identify eight different classroom setups. Each of these room setups has a specific purpose. Based on the type of lesson presentation, an instructor may need to set up the room several times during a class session. Let's look at how these rooms are used by instructors.

CLASSROOM-STYLE SETUP

Tables and chairs are facing in one direction toward the instructor's table or lectern. This style is frequently used when students are taking lecture notes or taking a written examination. This room setup does not encourage active student participation. Students sit back in their chairs, take notes, observe the instructor, and answer occasional questions.

DISCUSSION PRESENTATION SETUP

There are actually five different discussion-style setups identified in Figure 7-2. Those five styles are

1. Theater (large-group discussion)
2. Boardroom (independent work group)
3. Small-group discussion (independent work groups)
4. Discussion circle (large-group discussion)
5. Conference room (large-group discussion with AV aids)

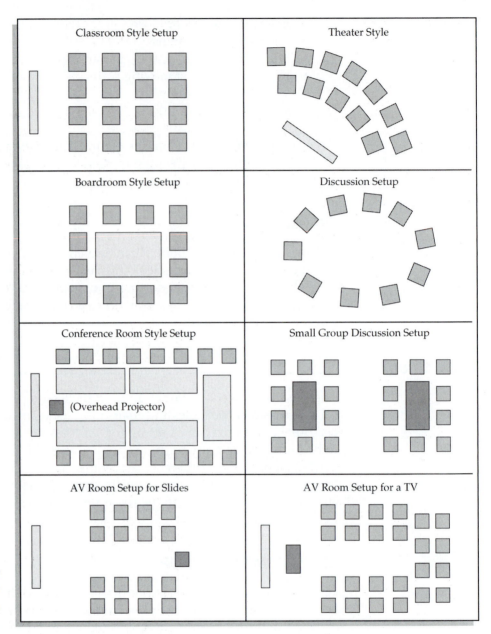

Figure 7-2
The eight different
types of classroom
setups.

Theater Style

This setup is designed for an instructor to present material, while being able to interact with the students. In a traditional classroom, students can "hide" behind other students, and an instructor loses sight of some students (Figure 7-3). The theater-style setting might be complemented with soft lighting to create a relaxed atmosphere. For presentations that deal with an informal subject, this style of setup is perfect. It also can be used for demonstrations, providing the material presented is large enough for everyone to see.

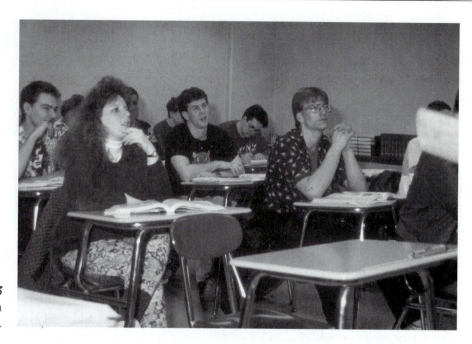

Figure 7-3
Traditional classroom
setup.

Boardroom Style

The boardroom style is ideal for lessons requiring an abundance of student interaction (Figure 7-4). Independent group discussions are frequently set up in this classroom style. Soft lighting helps to relax the students and encourages the group discussion. It is not effective in large groups because the length or width of the table defeats the purpose of the student interaction.

Small-Group Discussions

This is an adaptation of the boardroom-style setup. The exception is that there is more than one table, or there can be no tables. An entire class can be divided into small groups and assigned tables. This type of setup encourages independent group activities or can be used for tabletop models. When students are divided into practice groups, the classroom is divided into small practice groups without tables. The outdoor classroom activities too can be divided into specific group activities. Take for example a vehicle rescue evolution (Figure 7-5). One group of students can be the rescue personnel, while another group is the EMS crew. These are all examples of small-group activities that require the instructor to plan the activity based upon the classroom setup.

Discussion Circle

In this setup, the students move their chairs into a large circle and discuss topics for which there may be no definitive answer. Value questions are often used for this type of discussion setup.

Conference Room Setup with AV Aids

A final discussion style is the conference room setup, which encourages large-group interaction. This setup is frequently used for demonstrations or when AV aids are being used, especially the overhead projector. Students

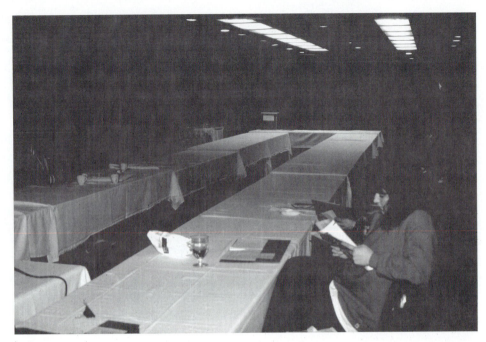

Figure 7-4
Boardroom style
setup.

are free from any obstructions, like other students' heads, while being able to have a face-to-face discussion. Soft lighting adds to the effect that this type of room setup can provide.

AUDIOVISUAL ROOM SETUP

There are numerous ways to set up a classroom for an AV aid presentation. Three examples were provided in the previous diagrams: one of them was the conference room setup; the other two are for slide presentations and for

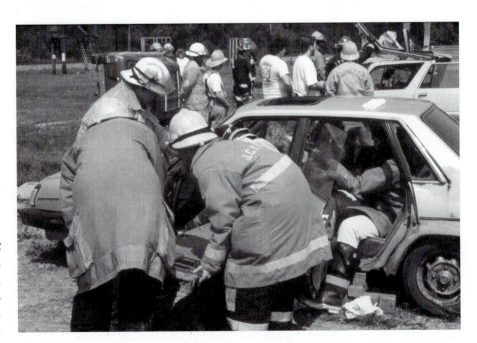

Figure 7-5
A rescue scenario
with an EMS team
and a rescue team is
an example of a
small-group setup.

TV presentations. All are examples of how a room may be set up so everyone can see the program material. Instructors should remember to make sure everyone can see and hear the material.

BREAKOUT ROOMS

Not shown in the diagram, many training institutes have more than one classroom available for an instructor to use. Smaller rooms are extremely useful for practice sessions. Breakout rooms tend to be less noisy than a classroom with all the students practicing at the same time. For examination purposes, breakout rooms become a prerequisite.

A point that has been stressed throughout this book is that any lesson material, even the room setup, eventually relates back to the lesson plan and the behavioral objectives. Instructors need to pay attention to room details if they wish to have a quality program. The equipment inside the room is as important as the room setup and environment.

COMPUTER LAB

Computer-based programming and Internet access are needed in many training programs. Textbooks include CD-ROMs and Internet addresses that contain program and supplemental information. Universities, trade schools, vocational-technical schools, and high schools have invested in setting up computer lab rooms. Instructors should attempt to gain access to these computer resources. Ideally, students should have access to computers in today's and tomorrow's classrooms.

Room Etiquette

Regardless of the room setup, there are rules of room usage that are followed. Following these common sense room rules will save an instructor a lot of complaints from fellow instructors, students, and maintenance staff.

1. Make sure that there are enough chairs and tables for the students. The instructor should make sure that the chairs are suitable for adult learners. Kindergarten size chairs do not work for large adult learners!
2. Once a room has been used, it should be straightened up for the next instructor. Students should police the classroom area before they are dismissed. It is a lot easier to have 20 students picking up the training equipment and refreshment containers than for the instructor to spend 20 minutes after class cleaning up the room. **NEVER** leave a room in worse shape than when you found it. If possible, it should be in better shape than you found it.
3. Have the room set up prior to the students arriving. This helps to maximize the actual classroom contact hours.

No-Wall Classrooms

What will tomorrow's classrooms look like? Formal classroom facilities are expensive to build and maintain. More and more educational materials are available via electronic media. Universities and training entities are offering courses via the Internet, CD-ROM, or by satellite. These "no-wall classroom" courses allow students to complete training at home, usually at a time when it suits the student.

Not all courses can be taught by these electronic methods. For skill-based programs, a formal classroom environment with a "live" instructor will still be required. Traditional classroom environments will likely include increased computer access points as more electronic educational resources are developed for emergency service courses.

Summary

Not every classroom has a traditional classroom setup. Emergency service instructors frequently use outside and specialty classrooms. These classrooms are no-wall environments that are effective for training emergency service personnel.

Instructors will find that every type of classroom has its own share of distractions. From rooms being too cold or too hot or having other classes' students loitering outside your classroom door during breaks to the banging of a construction site next door to your classroom, all can be classroom distractions. Instructors should try to control those distractions that they can and adapt their presentations around those that they cannot.

Chapter 8

Teaching Strategies and Methods

> ➤ OBJECTIVES

- Compare and contrast the inductive and deductive teaching strategies.
- Identify how the teaching strategy affects what teaching approach is used to present lesson material.
- Identify and describe various teaching methods.
- Describe the role of oral questions and how they affect the teaching method that is being used.
- Compare the various methods of instruction and identify the strengths and weaknesses of each method.
- Identify how an instructor selects the method of instruction for a particular subject.

How should an instructor present the lesson plan material? A variety of factors influence how an instructor uses a lesson plan. These factors have been outlined in previous chapters. Two factors, an instructor's personality characteristics and philosophical beliefs, are not influenced by external factors. These characteristics and beliefs are unique to individual instructors.

Let's look at an analogy, the instructional suitcase (Figure 8-1). It is time to go on vacation. After looking in several closets, the suitcase is located in the storage area. Dust is blown off and it is cleaned up. Clothes are selected and packed into the suitcase. So, what clothes are packed? Are they clothes used for cleaning and painting? Likely they are the best fitting, most attractive, and most comfortable clothes that are owned. Instructors select and use teaching methods that they feel comfortable with. This chapter looks at strategies and methods of instruction. Some of the teaching methods are going to feel comfortable, while other methods are going to be tight and simply will not fit. YOU will need to determine the methods of instruction that fit who you are.

Teaching Strategies

In simple terms, a teaching strategy is the approach used to present the lesson material. The process, or manner, an instructor actually uses to teach material is called the method of instruction, which is discussed later in this chapter.

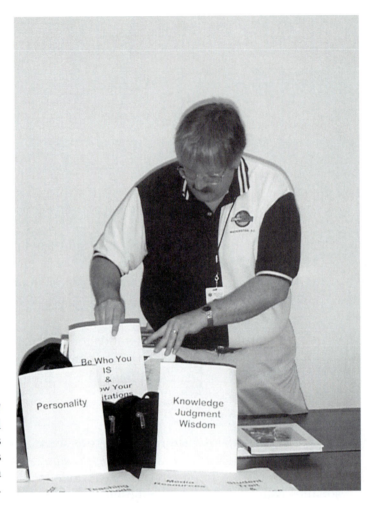

Figure 8-1
This instructional
suitcase contains
a variety of ways
to present lesson
material.

Two teaching strategies used by instructors are:

1.   Deductive strategy
2.   Inductive strategy[1]

DEDUCTIVE STRATEGY

When using a deductive strategy, the instructor provides the lesson material and states the lesson's conclusions for the students. The students are passive participants. The instructor does the work for the students. This strategy is useful when there are a large number of items to cover and there is limited time to present the material. The instructor presents the material and the students sit and absorb the lesson material.

Is it effective? It may be a practical way to present the material. It really depends upon the behavioral objectives, the type of students, and the personality characteristics of the instructor. The deductive strategy does not actively involve the students in the learning process. Students will not

[1]Pennsylvania Department of Health. *Rescue Instructor Curriculum* (Harrisburg, Penn.: 1988)

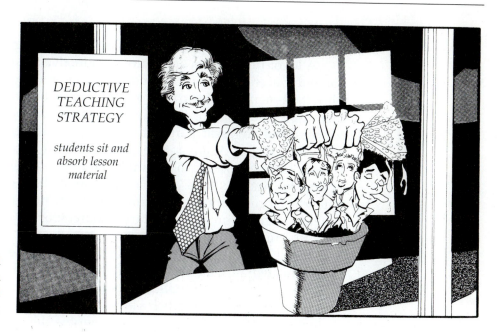

Students are asked to absorb the lesson material as presented by the instructor.

likely retain the same level of information as when they are actively involved in a presentation.

INDUCTIVE STRATEGY

This strategy relies upon active student involvement and minimal instructor input. Also known as the discovery approach, students are provided with minimal instructor input. Students research the material and develop their own conclusions. The instructor provides guidance and assistance to the students. The instructor facilitates and coordinates the learning environment.

Students do not become educational sponges, soaking up the instructor's information. Instead students do the research and find their own conclusions. The students are active participants in the learning process and retain more information because they are experiencing the learning. The inductive strategy closely follows John Dewey's concept of "learning by doing."[2]

What is the instructor's role in the inductive strategy? Primarily the instructors become facilitators. They will offer students constructive comments and encourage them when things seem to get bogged down. An instructor needs to ask critical questions to stimulate discussions. By the end of the lesson, the students must reach or exceed the lesson's objectives. The inductive strategy is dynamic and encourages students to research and potentially identify new ideas or techniques. Instructors who use this approach must be adaptable to these alternative concepts. If a student's conclusion is not identified in the lesson plan, that does not mean it is not acceptable. Instructors who use the inductive teaching strategy must be

---

[2]John Dewey, *Democracy & Education: An Introduction to the Philosophy of Education* (New York: MacMillan, 1930).

well versed in current research concepts. They also must be adaptable to new paradigms discovered when using this teaching strategy.

A lot of preparation goes into an inductive session. Reference books, computer access, equipment, and any other resources needed to accomplish the assignment are to be provided for the students. Instructors should plan to set aside a lot of classroom time. Time will be needed for students to access and do research in libraries or computer labs.

The principle disadvantage of the inductive strategy is the amount of classroom time required to accomplish the lesson assignment. It takes a lot of time for students to research and formulate their conclusions. Unfortunately, most curriculums and training institute instructor schedules do not provide adequate time or monetary resources for instructors to conduct extensive inductive training sessions.

Together, these two instructional strategies present a unique paradox. The inductive approach actively involves the students and promotes a higher retention of information. It requires an increased amount of classroom time for students to reach a lesson plan's conclusions. Meanwhile, the deductive strategy does not actively involve the students and results in poor to moderate retention of the lesson plan information. Yet the deductive strategy is efficient in its use of classroom time. So, where does an instructor find a balance between the strategies? One way to find a balancing point is to use a variety of teaching methods and try to blend the concepts of both strategies.

Teaching Methods

During a presentation, an instructor will use a variety of teaching methods. An instructor blends the methods together to make a presentation that is exciting, motivating, and informative. To be able to blend teaching methods, an understanding of each of the following pure methods is required. Each method has its own unique uses. Knowing when to use each method is critical.

LECTURE

By far, the lecture is the most frequently used and abused teaching method (Figure 8-2). Many students have an expectation when they enter a classroom (the students' paradigm); they expect the instructor to provide them with the lesson material. Many instructors feel compelled to use the lecture method for presenting the majority of the course material. Unless an instructor uses a mixed instructional method approach, the students' initial expectations will be met and often set the tone for an entire course.

Instructors who use the pure lecture method present facts, terms, and general information on a particular subject. The lecture method is the method most closely associated with the deductive strategy. The students are passive participants. Instructors often use the dry image board or an overhead transparency to emphasize important points, but for the majority of the presentation, the students sit and listen to the information. Using this

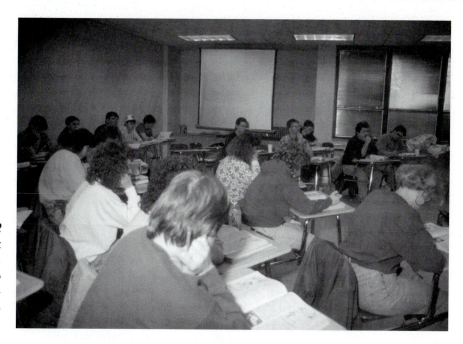

Figure 8-2
Lectures need not be a boring event. Instructors need to animate their presentations to keep a student's interest.

pure lecture approach, an instructor can expect about 20 percent retention of the information.[3]

Rarely do instructors use a pure approach. Successful instructors use the lecture method as a stepping-stone into their presentation. To increase the retention of the information, students need to become active participants within the lesson presentation. Educational resources, such as overheads, slides, videotapes, computer programs and simulations, and other multimedia aids improve the students' retention. Successful instructors roam through a classroom and encourage student interaction. They ask challenging oral questions and incorporate crossovers between pure lecture and other instructional methods, such as guided discussion.

GUIDED AND UNGUIDED DISCUSSION

The guided and unguided discussion formats are closely associated with the inductive teaching strategy. An instructor acts as both a facilitator and as a moderator in the discussion formats.

The guided discussion requires instructors to moderate discussion, and they often become participants in the discussion. Often, the instructor plays the role of the "devil's advocate" to stimulate the discussion and guide it along. The instructor can steer the students toward the desired outcome. The instructor should use predeveloped questions to stimulate discussion among the students.

There are two reactions that an instructor should be ready for. First, if there is no discussion, the instructor must be able to switch to an alternate

---

[3]Pennsylvania Department of Health. *Rescue Instructor Curriculum* (Harrisburg, Penn.: 1983).

teaching method. Often students are flat and simply do not want to participate in a group discussion. The second reaction is that the students become
so involved in the discussion that they end up getting off track discussing
unrelated issues. The instructor must intervene and refocus the discussion
onto the topic that should be discussed. New instructors prefer the guided
discussion because they have control over the lesson presentation. This differs from the next approach, the unguided discussion.

The unguided discussion is also called the discovery approach. It is
closely associated with the pure form of the inductive teaching strategy. As
is inferred from the word *discovery,* students seek out their own answers to
a lesson's questions. The instructor provides students with broad objectives
to solve. The students' task is to research, ask questions, and find the answers. Throughout the process, the instructor facilitates informational resources for the students. The instructor remains a nonparticipant in the
discussion. Only if the students reach a critical point in their discussion that
warrants the instructors' input will they get involved. The instructor freely
roams from group to group, monitoring the students' interaction. The
instructor acts as a third-party reviewer of the material and judges the students' presentations. The students are the active participants and the instructor assumes a passive role in the learning process.

Some instructors express reservations about using this approach.
These instructors are not comfortable using the unguided approach because they perceive a lack of control over the lesson material. Actually there
is a lot of control built into this approach. Instructors need to be more aware
of the material that is being researched and presented than they do when
they are the chief presenter. The instructor must be able to judge the content of the student's presentation and assure it meets the lesson plan's objectives. The instructor does a lot of preplanning, research, and construction
of discussion questions before the lesson is conducted.

The guided or unguided discussion approaches allow students to be actively involved in the lesson presentation. The more involved students become in a lesson, the better the learning experience becomes for the students.

SMALL GROUPS

Often used as part of an unguided discussion, dividing students into small
learning groups (from four to six students) allows students to actively participate in the learning experience. Small groups can be used for discussions and other classroom activities that require students to reach a
consensus decision.

How do you set up and use small groups? An instructor must create
clear and concise objectives. A time frame needs to be set for the group to
resolve the issues being discussed. Make sure to have on hand any educational resources or other materials that the group may require. A "mission
statement" or "purpose statement" for each group shall state the directions
the group is to follow. A timekeeper can keep the time for each group or use

a clock that all the groups can see. Once the small group activity begins, the instructor's role is to monitor each group's activities. When the time expires, the instructor should conduct a debriefing session. A spokesperson from each group should present the findings and results of the group. Following all of the groups' final presentations, the instructor should offer final outcomes from the activity.

An idea to encourage student participation in group activities is to offer some form of reward or recognition. Rewarding student participation in small group activities can help assure continued student participation in future group activities. The rewards do not need to be overly expensive or complex. An acknowledgement by the instructor of outstanding participation by a group of students can be enough to insure future student participation.

DEMONSTRATIONS

Students are impressionable. How an instructor initially presents a skill or piece of equipment often will determine how students will associate its use during practice sessions. Making this initial impression is called making referent contact. The use of demonstrations in training programs is more than just show-and-tell. There is a lot of planning and preparation that goes into a demonstration to get it right the first time.

The instructor must make referent contact, showing the students what is to be learned. If the skill demonstration is to assemble and use a hydraulic power tool, the entire skill is shown at full speed without interruption. It should look like it is expected to be in real life situations. The full demonstration is then followed up by a step-by-step review of the performance steps used to perform the skill.

Before conducting a demonstration, all of the students need to be able to see the demonstration. Small items may not be suited for a large-group demonstration; thus small-group demonstrations may be required. Have the equipment prepared before the demonstration. If assistant instructors are helping, practice performing the demonstration before doing it in front of the class.

Demonstrations bring real-life equipment and techniques directly in front of the students (Figure 8-3). The demonstration can use either a deductive or an inductive approach. The initial presentation is usually deductive, but as the step-by-step demonstration is presented, inductive concepts can be included.

Steps for conducting a demonstration include:

1. Prepare the equipment and arrange the demonstration area so everyone can see the presentation.
2. Introduce the skill by displaying the equipment that will be used in the demonstration. Explain to the students what to look for during the presentation.
3. Perform the demonstration completely and without interruption at full speed, as it would be done in real life.

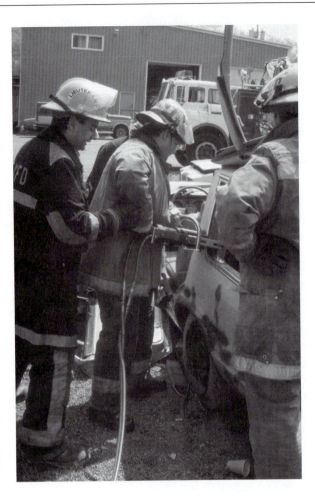

Figure 8-3
Assistant instructors
play a key role in
assuring students
perform the skills
correctly following
a demonstration.

4. Following the full presentation, perform the same demonstration using a step-by-step approach. Include students' questions and their comments at this point.
5. Clean up the demonstration area and continue with the classroom activities.[4]

The students take the information learned from the demonstration and will mimic their skill performance from the model presented by the instructor. The instructor must assure correct information is provided to the students, otherwise students will not correctly perform a skill. Students must be able to see the correct way to perform the skill if they are to have a positive contact referent to use when practicing a skill.

A videotaped presentation can be used for the introduction of a complete skill performed at full speed. Creative enhancements like patient actors and realistic surroundings can be included. The instructor performing a live step-by-step demonstration of the skill follows this taped presentation. Combining the taped presentation with a live demonstration can be an effective technique for presenting a demonstration.

---

[4]Pennsylvania Department of Health. *Rescue Instructor Curriculum* (Harrisburg, Penn.: 1988)

FIELD TRIPS

If instructors cannot bring real-life situations to the classroom, then they should take the classroom to the real-life situations. It is difficult to bring wrecked cars into an indoor classroom, and for practicing rescue skills, outdoor settings are required.

Field trips allow students to experience real-life experiences in controlled settings. Emergency service programs rely upon the use of field settings for many of their training program activities (Figure 8-4). The instructor needs to prepare the students for the field trip. Specific goals that will be accomplished during the field trip need to be identified. Special times, travel arrangements, equipment movement, rest room facilities, and meal arrangements must be taken into account. Drinking water and other fluid replacement solutions need to be included in outdoor training sessions.

The instructor needs to become a logistical engineer to effectively use a field trip. As explained in Chapter 7, unofficial training sites that are used (e.g., normal houses or rock cliffs) need to be carefully inspected for potential hazards. Training equipment needs to be moved and set up prior to the students arriving. Other arrangements, food, water, rest rooms, and student travel arrangements need to be made before a trip is conducted. Sufficient assistant instructors to supervise the activities are to be identified and the instructors briefed on their duties during the outdoor sessions. Unless the instructor takes care of the logistical details, a less-than-effective learning experience will result.

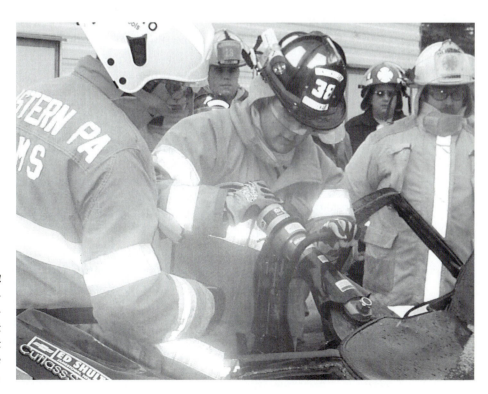

Figure 8-4
Field trips may require extensive logistical planning, but result in a significant learning experience for the students.

ROLE PLAYING

Emergency service training programs are excellent settings for the use of role-playing sessions. A role-playing session includes either the instructor or a student, or various students, acting out a predeveloped presentation. The script identifies specific wording that each participant should use during the presentation.

The instructor develops the script to fit into the lesson plan material. Instead of the instructor using a lecture or discussion technique to involve students, the role-playing session provides the same content material delivered by a lecture, but the students become the presenters of the material.

The script identifies the words that each person should be saying. It also includes the body movements, clothing that may be worn, various props, and the physical surroundings for the situation. A role-playing session can become a realistic learning experience for the students. They become active participants in the lesson presentation, and the instructor becomes a resource for the students' interpretation of the script. To be effective, students should have sufficient time to review and practice the script. Various groups of students can be given different role-playing scripts. Then the students can present the role-playing presentations to each other.

Role playing is not appropriate for every subject. But many topics like radio communication, scene control, legal presentations, and interpersonal communication are excellent for role-playing sessions. When instructors develop the lesson plan material, they should identify topics that could be used for role playing. The more planning and preparation an instructor puts into a role-playing script, the better the learning experience will be for the students.

The following is a role playing example:

Chief: Chief 42 to communications (anxious sounding).
Communications: Go ahead, Chief 42 (monotone response).
Chief: On location of a fully involved two-story structure fire. The fire's in both floors and it's spreading into adjacent buildings.
Communications: Okay, Chief 42. Do you request additional fire units in addition to Companies 42, 36, EMS 22, and Police 122?
Chief: Respond Companies 20, 33, and Chief 2 to this scene.
Communications: Received, Chief 42. Communications to Companies 20, 33, and Chief 2, respond to a structure fire assisting Chief 42.

The scenario can progress from this point to have additional students acting out the roles of the responding units. Then, simulated scene communications at the fire scene are acted out. Students become the chief officer, the communications dispatcher, and the emergency responders to the simulated fire scene. With realistic props, like working portable radios and surroundings, students can experience the feelings that Chief 42 and other responders are experiencing in the script.

Closely associated with role playing are simulations. The major difference between the two is that a role-playing presentation is scripted. The simulation is not scripted and the students control their own actions and feelings for a situation.

SIMULATIONS

Simulations are "instructor-created environments" that students are asked to perform various skills to solve problems. The simulation differs from a role-playing session because it does not use a script. Instead, the simulation uses a scenario. In Chapters 10 and 13, scenarios are discussed in detail. For this section's discussion, a scenario provides the students with a basic oral description of a scene.

> *You and your partner are dispatched to a back alley. Police have secured the scene. You find a twenty-year-old male who has been assaulted and is lying face down.*

The scenario provides the instructor with vital-sign information for the simulated patient actor. The makeup, moulage, props, and patient programming are identified. Specific treatments, equipment to be used, and the evaluation components are included in the scenario.

Using a scenario brings an entire learning experience together for a student. The knowledge and skills that have been presented throughout a program are incorporated into a simulation. Realism concepts add to the impact attained from the simulation.

In Chapter 13, simulation examples are expanded upon and realistic concepts are discussed. A scenario is a highly interactive learning tool. The instructor sets up the scenario and the students respond to it. Students learn by doing, and a simulation provides the students with that opportunity for learning by doing. Done correctly, a simulation can be as close to the "real thing" as one can get.

GAMES

Students can be motivated to learn material if they can enjoy their learning experience. Games provide a way for an instructor to present lesson material, using a nontraditional approach, which adds amusement to the learning experience. Learning and having fun doing it are ingredients for a positive learning experience.

Are we talking computer games? Not exactly, though computer games and simulations are discussed in Chapter 12. What is being discussed in this section are instructor-designed or commercially made games. Crossword puzzles, word searches, Trivial Pursuit, and offshoots of other board games like Jeopardy, Concentration, and Scrabble are examples of games that are used.

Games actively involve the students. For review sessions, instead of repeating the lecture material, use a game to review the same material.

Competition between different groups of students adds to the game. Learning becomes fun, and this motivated activity encourages students to participate and learn the material at the same time.

An entire program cannot be all fun and games, but an instructor needs to plan activities to encourage student participation. Using different games throughout a course can help students learn and retain information. It is just another way to teach lesson material.

INDEPENDENT STUDY

Different from any of the previous methods that have been discussed, independent study is designed around the individual students. Independent study has a specific assignment for an individual student to complete. Similar in design to the discovery approach, the students work by themselves on an assigned project and present their findings to the class. Classroom time can be set aside for having students work on independent study projects. This concept works especially well for computer learning stations, where it is just the computer and the student that are interacting. Many students are intimidated when working with other students and work better on their own. Independent study allows these students to work on their own and develop answers to study questions posed by the instructor.

The instructor acts as a resource center for students doing independent studies. Only when the students present the material does the instructor provide input. An instructor needs to observe and ask questions of students conducting independent studies to assure that they are not moving away from the lesson material.

Independent study has its limitations like other methods, however. Not every subject is conducive to this method, so instructors need to identify subjects that can be taught via the approach and incorporate this

An instructor does not have to be a super instructor to teach. Using the inductive approach is an alternative.

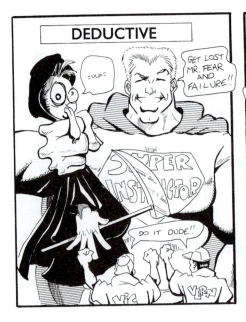

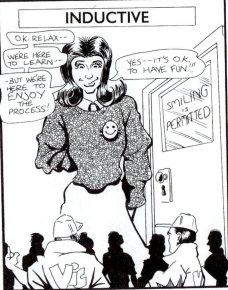

method into their presentations. The independent study method may be blended into a presentation using the lecture, demonstration, and guided discussion methods.

DISTANCE LEARNING

Via computers or video/audio systems, classrooms miles apart are being taught simultaneously. There are various levels of distance learning. These include:

- Satellite receivers
- Two-way audio
- Two-way audio and video
- Combination of video, telephone, or the Internet access
- Internet collaboration

Distance learning with video and audio allows the lead instructor to broadcast the presentation to one or more locations. Each receiving location usually has a local instructor/facilitator. Following the broadcast, the local instructor can conduct hands-on activities or answer questions about the presentation. In two-way learning systems, students can ask questions of the lead instructor. This form of distance learning is much more expensive than other forms of distance learning, such as Internet collaboration sessions.

Urban, suburban, and rural training sites can benefit from this type of teaching. This approach requires a commitment of the training institute and instructional personnel. There are significant initial and recurring costs. These costs must be factored into the use of this teaching approach.

EXPERIENTIAL LEARNING

Most adult learners have amassed a lot of lifetime learning experiences. Instructors can use these experiences to their advantage. They can tap into these experiences and build their lesson presentations around the students' experiences.

Instead of using predeveloped role-playing scenarios, ask students to reenact past events in their lives. Perhaps several students have experienced the sensation of being involved in an automobile accident. Ask them to share their thoughts, impressions, memories, and their overall experience of the accident.

Experiential learning utilizes the three educational learning domains, cognitive, affective, and psychomotor. An instructor who uses experiential learning must be prepared for the unexpected. One student's experience may be different from another. The instructor will need to facilitate discussion between the students and focus the students toward a conclusion.

Instructors select methods of instruction that they feel will present an informative yet motivational presentation. Many instructors try different methods of instruction each time they present a lesson, to improve their presentation style. Based on the teaching strategies, combined with educational studies that identify how students learn and retain information, the instructor selects the methods of instruction that are used in a presentation.

Oral Questions

Because oral questions are an immediate feedback mechanism, instructors can attain a feel for whether learning is occurring. For lectures, demonstrations, and guided discussions, an instructor must rely upon asking probing questions to stimulate discussions during the lesson presentation. When using oral questions, if an instructor does not ask a question in a clear manner, or does not wait long enough for a student to answer the question, the reason for asking the question in the first place is often lost. When an instructor has to water down a question to get an answer, why did the instructor ask the question in the first place? If the students are not responding to questions, this may be telling the instructor that they do not know the answer. No response, a partial response, an incorrect response, and the correct response all tell the instructor information about whether learning is occurring. Instructors expect the students to answer every question that is asked. When they do not answer, the instructor assumes that the question was poorly worded and rephrases the question. Often an initial question may be poorly worded, but do not assume that every question needs to be restated and clues provided to the students. If students are not responding to simple knowledge questions, this should be an indicator to the instructor that there is a potential problem in the learning experience.

Oral questions are formed from four categories of oral questions:

- Recall (basic knowledge)
- Convergent (comprehension and analysis)
- Divergent (brainstorming / problem-solving)
- Value (beliefs, sensation, feelings)

Oral questions are designed to stimulate a response from the students. If students cannot answer recall-level questions, it is doubtful that divergent and value questions, which are higher-level questions, will be answered successfully. This is not to say that instructors should not ask these qualitative types of questions; they should. Divergent and value questions stimulate critical thinking.

To involve students, appropriate oral questions are needed to make a lecture presentation come alive. Oral questions often lead a lecture presentation into a guided discussion format. This type of method blending is a characteristic that successful instructors perform without extensive planning.

Instructors are not only using oral questions to stimulate classroom discussion, but they are also asking the questions to assess the quality of the learning experience. Oral questions provide instant feedback to an instructor. Instructors often use responses to the oral questions as their thermometer to the learning experience. Thus an instructor can use an oral question to stimulate a discussion and, at the same time, evaluate the students' response. Good oral questions both stimulate and evaluate. Combined, they enhance the learning experience for the students.

Summary

For each of the teaching strategies, adaptations can be identified. Because instructors use teaching approaches that match their personality characteristics, there are unlimited variations of the pure methods that are presented in this chapter. Every method of instruction has its strengths and weaknesses. A method that may work for one instructor may not work for another instructor. Even a lesson plan written for one group of students may not work for another group of students taught by the same instructor.

Methods of instruction are not just selected from material presented in this chapter. Rather, a method of instruction is selected from the material contained throughout this book. So many variables are factored into the selection of a method. A selection is made only after looking at who the instructor is, who the students are, the type of presentation, the time allotted to the presentation, the educational resources for the presentation, plus many more variables. All influence the selection of the method of instruction.

These factors are why successful instructors do so much preplanning before a presentation. Months of preparation go into developing a method of instruction. If an instructor is to become successful, he cannot expect to put a lesson presentation together overnight. Quality education comes from adequate planning and presenting. Instructors have a duty to provide the highest-quality educational experience possible. Selecting and using appropriate methods of instruction are part of providing quality educational experiences for emergency service personnel.

Chapter 9

Psychomotor Development

> ➤ **OBJECTIVES**

- Define *psychomotor skill.*
- Define *motor skill.*
- Identify the formula necessary for successful skill performance.
- State the importance of overlearning a skill and identify how it improves skill retention.
- Identify the role of task analysis in a skill presentation.
- Compare distributed practice with drill practice.
- Identify the taxonomy of the psychomotor domain.
- Review the development of a skill objective and the lesson plan.
- Identify the need to make referent contact before demonstrating a skill.
- Review the need to teach principles, not methods, during a skill development session.
- Identify the physical and mental characteristics that are required to perform a skill.
- Describe the steps involved in a skill presentation, with specific emphasis to be placed on the following:
  —Full skill demonstration
  —Step-by-step skill demonstration
  —Supervised and unsupervised practice sessions
  —Independent practice
  —Evaluation of the skill
- Identify the learning phases that students go through to master a skill.
- Identify a practice ethic for students learning a skill.
- Review the roles that instructors need to play during skill practice sessions.
- Identify the interpersonal communications needed between the instructor and the students during skill training sessions.
- State the role that assistant instructors play in successful skill development.
- Identify the prelogistics and postlogistics for setting up and teaching a skill station.
- Identify and define the role that realism plays in skill stations.
- Explore the use of a video camera for improvement in the skill performance.
- Explore the future use of computer interactive programming for improving a student's skill performance.

Performing skills are included in almost every emergency service training program. Students perform skills using learned material that is placed into motion. Being able to understand the material and coordinate appropriate body movements is a definition of psychomotor development (Figure 9-1).

Being able to perform a manual skill involves the integration of a series of mental and physical abilities. For example, to apply a traction splint involves motor abilities, knowledge, and interpersonal skills. This chapter looks at how an instructor develops both mental and physical skills. How a skill is taught and supervised by an instructor influences a student's performance. Students should be encouraged to reach the highest performance level that they are capable of attaining. The highest skill level is the mastery level. At this level students are confident and perform the skill with 100 percent accuracy. Attaining this level of skill proficiency requires time and unending support from the instructor.[1]

The Basics

In almost every chapter of this book, skill instruction has been mentioned. In Chapter 2, traits that a student must have to perform a skill were identified. An adult learner tends to be easier to instruct than high-school-aged students because adults have developed control of their motor abilities. High school students are developing their motor abilities and do not have realistic experiences to draw upon. An instructor must prepare a skill presentation with these concerns in mind.[2] In Chapter 3, the importance of the instructor being the role model for demonstrating the skill and being the coach for the students was identified. The instructor teaches skills by principles, instead of methods. *Principles* are the basic components of a skill. Principles rarely change. Conversely, *methods* are variable and are dynamic. For example, in the case of opening a jammed door, the principle would be to safely remove or open the door without causing further injury to a victim, while minimizing the time and effort upon the rescuers. The methods to accomplish this task range from the use of a power hydraulic spreading tool to the use of a wrecking bar. A key point from this chapter looks at personality traits of an instructor or assistant instructor and how they influence a student's performance.[3] Positive reinforcement is needed if learning is to occur.[4]

Chapter 4 looked at skills from a different viewpoint. Educational psychologists provided various theories and explanations on how skills are performed. A skill consists of not just a motor component (motor skill or the psychomotor domain), that is, where a student actually performs physical

[1]Anita J. Harrow. *A Taxonomy of the Psychomotor Domain* (New York: David McKay, 1972).

[2]Ibid.

[3]Thomas Good and Jere Brophy. *Educational Psychology: A Realistic Approach* (New York: Holt, Rinehart, and Winston, 1977).

[4]Robert N. Singer. *Motor Learning and Human Performance*, 3rd ed. (New York: Macmillan, 1980).

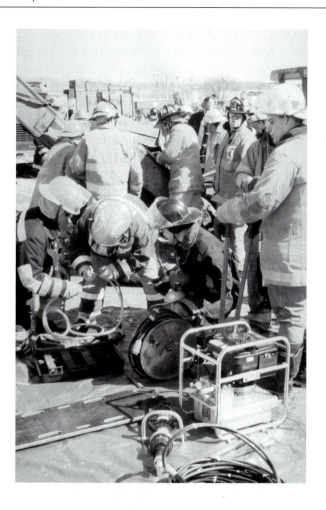

Figure 9-1
Assembly of rescue
equipment.

tasks; a student must have knowledge (cognitive domain) of why and how he is to perform the skill. The last component of a skill involves the attitude, feelings, or motivation displayed by the student (affective domain). A skill involves the interaction of these three learning domains. When teaching a skill, an instructor should provide an atmosphere for students to attain all three components.[5]

How to create a skill lesson plan was discussed in Chapter 5. The psychomotor domain helps an instructor to look at the physical and mental abilities that are required to perform the skill. A task analysis helps the instructor determine exactly how to perform the skill by breaking the skill into its components. The lesson plan is not based only on these components, but it uses behavioral objectives to identify the overall skill. Then in Chapters 6 and 7, how students' skill performance can be enhanced by their surroundings is discussed. For example, using a video camera can improve students' skill performance by allowing them to see themselves performing the skill. A prerequisite for any skill is to have enough space to practice the skill. Chapter 7 explains the types of facilities that enhance skill training. Chapters beyond this one provide additional information about skills.

---

[5]Harrow, 1972.

In Chapter 10, skill assessments are reviewed. Chapter 12 examines how computer technology can improve skill performance. Chapter 13 reviews the use of realism concepts. Making the skill realistic is a crucial part of successful skill performance.

Each of these chapters deals with some component in the development, instruction, enhancement, and evaluation of a skill. Remaining portions of this chapter will build upon the basics identified in these chapters.

The Skill Formula

Good skill performance does not happen by accident. Practice does not make a skill perfect by itself; additional components are required. What is needed to perform a skill? The answer lies within this skill formula:

$$\text{Skill} = \text{Speed} + \text{Accuracy} + \text{Form} + \text{Adaptability}[6]$$

The speed at which a skill is practiced influences how it will be performed. "Full speed ahead" should be the motto that instructors use when teaching a skill. Students should practice a skill at a rate that is as close to real-life speed as is possible. While performing the skill at full speed, it should be performed correctly. It is of little benefit to rapidly perform a skill incorrectly. While increasing the performance of the skill, the accuracy in performing the skill should also be improved, or at least maintained.

How do students perform the skill? Are they all thumbs? Are they nervous wrecks? Do they appear confident? Or are they cocky and arrogant while performing the skill? Do they make it look easy, or does it look like they are in distress while performing the skill? These questions involve the form component. If this was Olympic ice skating, the form component of the skill would be equivalent to the artistic impression component of ice skating. Any of these questions can be asked when evaluating the form component. Skills should be performed with ease and should not seem to use a lot of energy.

The final component is adaptability. Emergency scenes are ever changing. One second a fire is contained to the living room, the next it is racing up the stairs to the second floor. Students need to be able to demonstrate adaptability when they are faced with a situation that may not be like the textbook model. Students should be given opportunities to adapt a skill to a less than ideal setting in a training session.

When a student can exhibit speed + accuracy + form + adaptability, the result is a successful skill performance. When one or more of the components are out of balance, this will affect the overall performance of the skill. When teaching a skill station, look for these four variables. Assess how the students are performing the skill and identify which components are in need of improvement.

---

[6]Singer, 1980.

Student Personality Traits

Factors that are indirectly included in the skill formula and have an effect on the performance of a skill are the student's personality characteristics. Here are the dominant traits:

1. Body build
2. Motor abilities
3. Physical ability (strength)
4. Personality
5. Interpretation ability
6. Intelligence
7. Emotions
8. Fear
9. Attitude
10. Aspirations/goals
11. Specific skills
12. Age
13. Sex
14. Sense acuity

Many more traits can be added to this list. The point is, a deficit in any of these factors can influence the performance of a skill. The instructor should be aware of any underlying deficits that might result in poor performance. If an entire class is performing the skill poorly or incorrectly, the method of instruction should be reviewed.

Preskill Setup

Skill presentations require extensive preparation on the part of an instructor. From the classroom environment to the training equipment, all need to be ready before the class begins. The lesson plan provides most of the logistics for the lesson presentation. Still, actually setting up equipment, preparing lesson materials, briefing and practicing the skill with assistant instructors, and preparing the classroom area for the session takes time.

When performing a skill, it is important to use as much realism as possible. The environment in which a skill is performed can affect the student's performance. Remember that adult learners do not relate well to unrealistic situations. As a part of their learning process, realistic situations need to be used whenever possible.

An essential part of the preskill preparation involves preparing the students. An explanation of the skill session should be conducted before the initial demonstration of a skill. Remember the concept of a referent contact. Students need to have some form of previous experience or knowledge to build upon. An oral explanation of the skill gives the students information to look for during the skill presentation.[7]

---

[7]Harrow, 1972.

Skill Lesson Presentation

The skill lesson plan identifies how the lesson is taught. Included within the lesson plan is a component called the *task analysis*, which explains how a student completes a skill. The task analysis identifies both mental images and physical movements that are used to perform a skill. The task analysis breaks a large skill into separate component parts. When writing a task analysis, an instructor should envision an individual who has no training. Each step of the skill must be clearly identified. With a well-written task analysis, a student should be able to practice and perform a skill.

So, how should an instructor teach a skill? The following are components used to teach skills:

1. Skill introduction/full instructor demonstration
2. Step-by-step instructor demonstration
3. Direct supervision of students practicing
4. Indirect supervision of students practicing
5. Independent student practicing
6. Evaluation of the student's skill performance[8]

SKILL INTRODUCTION/FULL INSTRUCTOR DEMONSTRATION

This is considered the most important phase of skill instruction. The instructor presents the skill at the speed and accuracy that is expected from emergency personnel in real-life settings. Students will remember how an instructor performed the skill. They will try to mimic the instructor's movements when they practice. If the skill was performed incorrectly by the instructor, chances are that the skill will not be performed correctly by some students.

Often, instructors skip over the full demonstration component and move onto the step-by-step demonstration. The students never see how the skill is supposed to look at real speed. The initial skill becomes a key reference for students. Doing it right the first time becomes essential, not just in education, but in real-life settings.

Doing the skill right the first time is not an easy task. Instructors must practice performing the skill before making the actual presentation. As suggested in Chapter 6, some instructors have produced videotapes of a skill performance or have used commercially made tapes of the skill presentation. It is essential to do the skill right the first time and not to leave the students with half an image of the skill, which can occur when presenting a skill using the step-by-step approach.

Introduce the skill presentation. For example, tell the students:

The assistant instructors and I will be demonstrating the rigging of a 3:1 mechanical advantage leverage system. Pay attention to the anchor points, the types of knots being used, and the main contact points on the object, which is being moved.

---

[8]Pennsylvania Department of Health. *Instructor Care* (Harrisburg, Penn.: 1988).

This type of introduction allows students to look for these behaviors during the full demonstration. It is important to indicate that if students have a question during the demonstration to wait until the end of the demonstration. It is quite possible that their question may be answered by seeing the entire skill presentation. But more important, a student's question during a full skill demonstration will interrupt the entire demonstration, thus destroying the impact of the demonstration.

Once the full demonstration begins, complete the demonstration without interruption. Many times an instructor will start demonstrating a skill and partway through will stop and begin providing commentary on the specific components of the skill. This defeats the purpose of performing a full demonstration. Do the full demonstration, either live or on tape, and then follow it up with a live, step-by-step demonstration. Using a two-step instructor demonstration first allows students to see how to perform the skill at "real-time speed," and then it shows them how the skill was actually performed.

STEP-BY-STEP DEMONSTRATION

Immediately following the full demonstration, the instructor should perform a step-by-step demonstration (Figure 9-2). The step-by-step demonstration breaks the skill down into its component parts. The presentation is much slower than the full demonstration. Students are encouraged to stop the instructor and ask specific questions regarding specific action steps.

The step-by-step demonstration should be a live presentation whenever possible. The instructor and student interactions are key ingredients in learning a skill. Students should be encouraged not to leave with any unanswered questions. If a student does not understand the skill components,

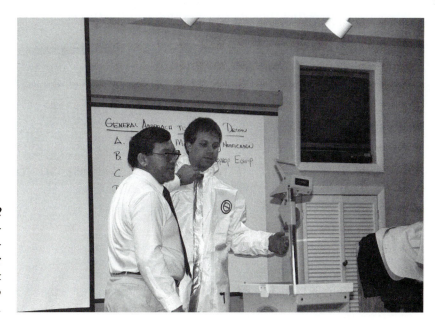

Figure 9-2
Immediately following a full demonstration, an instructor should conduct a step-by-step demonstration.

then the instructor should repeat the components that are being questioned. An unanswered question at this point may influence how a student performs the skill in the future.

The primary instructor and assistant instructors should perform the skill. Often, while the assistant instructors perform the skill, the primary instructor can give an oral description of the skill's components. This format allows the primary instructor to maintain a proper position in front of the students, while monitoring both the students and the assistant instructors.

SUPERVISED PRACTICE

The ideal time to start practicing a skill is immediately following the instructor's skill demonstration. Students are usually eager to learn the skill. Whenever possible, the instructor should plan the practice sessions in conjunction with the skill demonstration.

The practice sessions discussed in this section are centered on supervised sessions. Because students are eager to learn a skill, their desire to perform the skill will be high. However, their manual dexterity rarely results in perfect skill performance during the first practice session. Students are going to make errors. The instructors need to become coaches for the students. This is not the time or the place for criticism.[9] Instructors need to offer guidance and support, while they make note of the mistakes. Use an approach called "+ − +" to provide students with realistic feedback. Tell the students the skill components that were done correctly and incorrectly. Students need to have a knowledge of their results if they are to improve their skill performance.[10]

Often instructors ask the question, "When is a good time to stop the students to correct a mistake?" The answer is usually, "When the students have finished the skill presentation."[11] There is, of course, an exception: When an unsafe act will occur and cause potential injury to any of the participants. Stopping the students too soon may interrupt their learning process. Mistakes that they made are often caught and corrected by the students themselves. Students often need to fail, so that they can do the skill correctly the next time. The key role for an instructor is to provide the students with honest and sincere input, input that is balanced and constructive.

Must there be an instructor for every pair of students? The answer is no. For example, the U.S. Department of Transportation's National Standard Curriculum for EMTs suggests an instructor-to-student ratio of 1 to 6.[12] Other curriculums may have a 1-to-5 or 1-to-4 ratio, depending upon the type of training program activity.[13] An instructor should consult the curriculum being used by the training institute. Often there may be specific

---

[9]Good and Brophy, 1977.

[10]Singer, 1980.

[11]Robert Kerr. *Psychomotor Learning* (Philadelphia, Penn.: W. B. Saunders, 1982).

[12]U.S. Department of Transportation. *National Standard Correction for EMT Basic* (Washington, D. C.: 1994).

[13]Pennsylvania Department of Health. *Vehicle Rescue Curriculum* (Harrisburg, Penn.: 1999).

instructor-to-student ratios for a training institute. An instructor ratio might also be a part of the training institute's reimbursement system. Consult the training institute for specific student-to-instructor ratios for the particular program.

How the students practice the skill is important. Students practicing a skill need to work toward the speed and accuracy presented during the full demonstration. Students not actively practicing the skill need to be watching the other groups performing the skill. Seeing how other students perform a skill can enhance a waiting student's performance. The waiting students can use this time to mentally review how to perform the skill. Students should be able to form a mental image of how they will perform the skill.[14] Athletes use this technique to review a skill before they actually perform. This technique creates a positive image for the athletes. They picture themselves performing the skill correctly, which helps them to physically perform the skill.[15] Emergency personnel should use this technique before they perform a skill. Every step of the skill should be reviewed mentally before they actually perform the skill. Both the mental and physical phases of a skill need to be practiced.[16]

Practice alone does not mean that students will improve their skill performance. Knowledge of their results is an important element. A second element that is as important as the knowledge of their results is the format of the practice session. Rest periods interspersed between the practice sessions should be planned and practiced. Students get fatigued while performing skills. Interspersing rest periods between practice sessions helps to lessen the fatigue associated with performing a skill. Students who become fatigued begin to make errors. In the initial practice sessions, the instructor should closely monitor the students' physical abilities. Students who are making errors because they are fatigued and frustrated should be given an extended break. During the break, the instructor should help the students form mental pictures of how the skill should be performed. Being a coach means looking out for the student's best interests (Figure 9-3).[17]

Supervised practice sessions are important from a disciplinary perspective. Yes, from a disciplinary perspective! The instructor often needs to play the role of a drill sergeant. Students often use practice sessions for an extended break time. Time given for skill development is a precious asset. Instructors need to encourage students to make the best use of their practice time. One educational study[18] looked at the length of time given for practice sessions during CPR programs. The study determined that the amount of actual practice time for an individual student performing CPR was significantly less than the total time provided for the entire session. Instructors should encourage their students to make the most of any practice

---

[14]Singer, 1980.

[15]John D. Lawther. *The Learning and Performance of Physical Skills* 2nd ed. (Upper Saddle River, N. J.: Prentice Hall, 1977).

[16]Singer, 1980.

[17]Ibid.

[18]W. Kaye, et al. *Resuscitation*, vol. 21 (Limerick, Ireland: Elsevier Scientific, 1982), pp. 67–87.

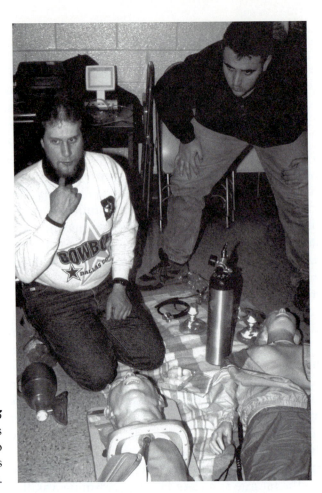

Figure 9-3
An instructor needs
to be present to
answer the student's
questions.

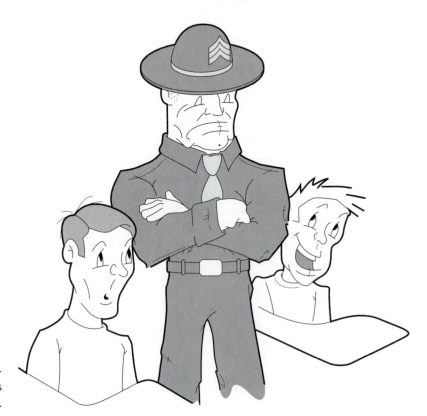

Drill sergeant watch-
ing over students
practicing.

session (Exhibit 9-1). Don the drill instructor's hat and encourage the students to practice the skill instead of having them talking about unrelated subjects or being wall decorations.

Words of caution: do not forget the assimilator learner. The assimilator type learner learns best by watching other students. A student who is not eagerly participating but is watching other students perform the skills may be learning. Be careful not to disrupt this learning experience. Get to know the students and find out, through their actions, which are the assimilator learners. They usually are not too difficult to identify.

Supervised practice sessions are important for assuring that the students understand the skills. Supervised practice is essential in the initial phases of a student's skill development. But for students to begin the climb to the mastery level of skill performance, they need to have less step-by-step instructor input and more independent practice time.

INDIRECT PRACTICE

Indirect practice is used after students have begun to perform a skill with improved accuracy and speed. For continued skill development, an instructor needs to allow the students to practice without an instructor directly looking over their shoulders. The instructor needs to become an observer of the classroom activities instead of watching individual groups of students.

For students who are having difficulty with a skill, an assistant instructor should provide individualized instruction. Meanwhile, the rest of the students can practice without a lot of individualized attention.

Provide the more advanced students with challenging situations. Allow them to experiment and adapt their skills to solve difficult scenarios.

Exhibit 9-1

Moderation for Skills

There is often a misconception associated with the highly motivated students in a class. Instructors often think that these overachievers will be the best students for performing a skill. Educational studies have found that the best students are those who are moderately motivated. During skill training, moderate to difficult tasks have been found to improve the student's overall performance. Moderation when performing a skill is a key for improving a student's performance.

Source: Robert Singer. *Motor Learning & Human Performance: An Application to Physical Education Skills,* 2nd ed. (New York: Macmillan, 1980).

Real-world settings are not textbook models. For example, fires are not just located on the first floor of a building. Fires often extend between the walls and ceilings of a building. What was a one-floor fire can become a two-story fire in minutes. Students practicing fire suppression techniques need to be able to spot fire extension locations and extinguish them. This type of experience comes from the instructor challenging the students to find the fire.

Safety remains a primary concern when teaching any skill. Instructors need to be even more cautious during these types of practice sessions. If an unsafe activity is about to be performed, the instructor has the responsibility to stop that skill activity.

INDEPENDENT STUDY SESSION

In Chapter 8, an independent study session was referenced to knowledge-oriented topics. But there is a role for an independent study session within a skill practice session. Instructors may wish to consider using an independent session, providing that the type of skill that is performed fits this approach. It would be tough for a pair of students to set up a burn building scenario, to operate the fire engine, to lay the hose lines, to gain entrance into the building, and to suppress the fire all by themselves. This would be unreasonable. But practicing mouth-to-mask ventilation on a training manikin may be an appropriate skill for independent skill practice.

Independent study allows a student to learn knowledge or skill subjects by themselves. After students have attained satisfactory performance in front of an instructor, they may be considered candidates for an independent study session. This type of session allows students to practice a skill on their own. The components of the skill—speed, accuracy, form, and adaptability—are enhanced and improved by the students as they try to better their overall performance.

Technology can be used to assist students improve their skill performance. During the independent skill session is an ideal time for the use of a stationary video camera. Students can videotape their performance. Then they can immediately review the tape and critique their own performance. The tape provides an independent record of their performance. As suggested in other chapters, the video camera can be used for students in other phases of their skill training. Another use would be for those students in a supervised practice session who are repeating the same mistakes over and over again. The video camera allows these students to visualize their performance. An instructor can pinpoint the areas that are done correctly and explain how to improve components that are being performed poorly. For independent study sessions and for students with learning difficulties, the use of a video camera should be considered an essential training adjunct.

The independent study approach is not for every student or class. Students must be able to demonstrate their desire to improve a skill for this type of approach to be successful. It is an approach that instructors may wish to use with the gifted students in their class. While other students are practicing their skill in a supervised setting, these gifted students can be using the independent study approach.

Independent study sessions are an alternative for many students. Instructors should consider using this type of activity in a presentation whenever the lesson material allows. Additionally, the level of student motivation will affect the use of this approach. For the motivated students, this approach will enhance their skill practice sessions.

EVALUATION

The goal of learning a skill is to be able to reach the mastery level of performance. This goal needs to be accurately assessed during a practical skill evaluation. As opposed to a pencil and pen test, students are to physically demonstrate the performance of a skill.

A skill evaluation session is designed to be a learning tool for the students. To become better at performing a skill, students need to know what to do to improve their performance. Athletes are always looking for ways to improve their skill performance. They strive to lower their performance time by another tenth of a second. They make the performance look easier than it really is. These same goals hold true for emergency service personnel. The skill evaluation becomes a benchmark for the students to see where they are at a given time and where they need to be.

Instructors can use two approaches to assess a skill. The two approaches are to look at either the process or the end product.[19] *Process* evaluation looks at a skill from a step-by-step component viewpoint. How well does a student perform components 1, 2, 3, and 4, and are they in the correct order? The *end product* evaluation looks at the skill performance from a broad perspective. How does a student use the skill components to solve the entire scenario? It does not grade the students as much on the specific 1, 2, 3, and 4 components. Critical performance standards are identified and measured. The two evaluation approaches should be used separately. The process evaluation approach is ideal for initial practice sessions. At the end of a course, the end process approach can be used to evaluate a student's overall ability to perform a skill in real-life settings.

Countless factors influence the students' performance during an examination. For instance, mention the word *exam* to some students and their anxiety levels rise to new heights. The educational setting often influences the students' performance. If the examination setting is not realistic and requires the students to imagine one that is realistic, the usefulness of the examination can be questioned. Adult learners need effective realism, not pretend settings.[20] Likewise, the scenario that is used must be appropriate. All these factors can influence a student's performance.

The skill examination is designed to assess the student's mastery of the skill. It is a valuable learning tool. Students need to have feedback as they learn a skill. A fair skill evaluation can provide a student with invaluable

---

[19]Pennsylvania Department of Health. *Rescue Instruction Curriculum* (Harrisburg, Penn.: 1988).

[20]Malcolm Knowles. *The Adult Learner: A Neglected Species* (Houston, Tex.: Gulf, 1990).

information about his overall performance. The evaluation should note both positive and weak aspects of a skill performance. The only way students will improve their performance is if they are provided with accurate input. This is coupled with a supportive coach (instructor) to provide the student with the assistance needed to improve. Often, these are not the usual purposes that students and instructors recall when discussing an examination. Yet these should be the reasons for evaluating a student's skill performance.[21]

Too often, practice sessions are geared toward what the students need to know for a certification examination. Instructors should prepare students for activities that they will use in the field. If students are taught to do it right in the field, they will likely do it right for an examination.

Practical examinations are tremendous educational resources. Instructors and students both benefit from the results. Good, bad, or neutral results do relate different types of information. Students need this information so they can continue to perform the skill correctly. Instructors act as their coaches. The instructor needs to be in the student's corner. Support from the instructor is essential for a student's success.

Overlearning and Drill Paradox

There is an interesting paradox in learning a skill.[22] After a student performs a skill correctly one time, the student goes into an overlearning phase. Overlearning is not bad. It tends to result in improved skill retention. But there is a point when overlearning becomes overkill. Students in overkill gain little or no growth from practice sessions. But how do students reach this point of diminished learning? Most commonly it is through the instructor's use of a continuous drill technique.

The concept of continuous practice sessions, such as drill sessions, causes overlearning to occur. The instructor has the students perform the skill over and over again, even when the skill is performed correctly. Drill can be useful for students up to a certain point.[23] But when a skill session becomes boring, little improvement will occur. Drilling students begins to cause errors, often due to the student's fatigue. Meanwhile, it can assist other students to improve their skill performance. This, of course, is the dilemma. Overlearning can improve the students' skill retention. Drilling students causes overlearning to occur. Both have a dangerous side effect. Both overlearning and drill take time away from other areas of learning. Going past the reasonable point of overlearning causes a decrease in learning instead of an increase. An instructor must recognize the signs of fatigue and modify the practice session to meet the students' abilities.

Ample practice time is essential for skill retention to be increased. Students need to be challenged in their training sessions. Improved performance is attained from harder goals than from easier ones. During a prac-

---

[21]Singer, 1980.
[22]Ibid.
[23]Lawther, 1977.

tice session, an instructor needs to drill and provide challenging situations for the students to solve. These concepts lead to productive overlearning and discourage overkill. Constructive encouragement from the coach goes a long way to improve the student's performance.

Interpersonal Communication

The instructor is the coach for the students. As a coach, both the good and poor aspects of a performance need to be identified. Students are not going to improve their performance unless they get objective information from their coach. Students need to build trust between themselves and their coach. If an instructor is not sincere and concerned about a student's performance, this trust will never develop. Building trust between the instructor and the students is what this section is about.

Successful athletic coaches are respected by their players. Respected coaches are able to communicate openly with their players. If the players perform incorrectly, the coach identifies the mistakes and identifies ways to correct the mistakes. When a game is lost, the successful coach does not yell at the players. Instead, the coach identifies areas that caused the players to lose and explains how they will not be defeated again. When the players are successful, the coach is there to give them their deserved praise. In addition, the coach is there to offer constructive comments to improve the players' performance.

Emergency service instructors need to become respected coaches during skill training sessions. It is very easy to revert to the "carping critic" or "task master" roles.[24] These roles offer little constructive support to students. Both these roles should be avoided when teaching a skill. Likewise, being a "cheerleader" or a "salesman" can be bad.[25] Telling the students only what they did correctly and not identifying the areas of poor performance can negatively affect the students' performance. An effective coach is able to objectively communicate both the positive and negative aspects of a performance. Students are only going to improve if they have an accurate knowledge of their performance.

An instructor's role is to be the coach and provide this information to the student. That is what effective interpersonal communications is all about. Honest and constructive comments will go a long way to provide positive reinforcement of a skill performance. The students need to depend upon the instructor to provide them with accurate information, especially during skill development. Mistrust and poor performance are often the trade-off in a classroom with poor interpersonal communication. Interpersonal communication is for all the students and instructors. Both the primary and assistant instructors need to encourage the students. Picking the assistant instructors can be a key component that influences how students will perform a skill.

---

[24]Good and Brophy, 1977.
[25]Ibid.

Assistant Instructors

Assistant instructors monitor large portions of practice sessions. With large classes, the primary instructor uses reliable assistant instructors. Together, both the primary and assistant instructors become the coaches for the students.

A lead instructor cannot supervise every group of students or every assistant instructor. Assistant instructors must be trusted to share similar information that the primary instructor would normally present. The assistant instructor should mirror the instructional style of the primary instructor.

What happens if an assistant instructor does not mirror the primary instructor? What results is a mismatch in teaching styles that leads to the students becoming confused. A statement such as, "But the primary instructor didn't tell us to do it that way," is commonly heard when a mismatch in teaching styles occurs. A similar statement can be heard when assistant instructors teach a variety of methods instead of basic principles. Both are associated with a mismatched instructional style. Instructors should use assistant instructors that reflect their teaching style. A supportive and caring primary instructor is meaningless if there is an overly critical assistant instructor working with the students.

Select the assistant instructors wisely. The following are criteria that might be used in the selection of an assistant instructor:

1. Possesses common teaching style with the primary instructor.
2. Demonstrates proficiency in performing skills, which he or she will be teaching.
3. Has minimum training at the level of instruction that he or she will be teaching (e.g., an EMT training an EMT).
4. Demonstrates desire to improve personal skill proficiency.
5. Is mature and exhibits positive role model characteristics.
6. Is motivated for the educational experience, not other intrinsic factors (e.g., ego, monetary reimbursement).
7. Is available for training sessions.
8. Demonstrates an understanding of instructional methods used to instruct skill sessions.
9. Is a respected emergency provider within his or her local area.

Item 8 is an aspect that cannot be overlooked. Just because assistant instructors can perform skills in a field setting does not mean that they can teach the skill in an educational setting. In other words, not every good field provider becomes a good instructor. Assistant instructors need to be exposed to formal teaching approaches used to teach skill sessions.

In the state of New York, the Department of Health identified a need to create a special course to train lab instructors. The lab instructors spend significant time with students and are the individuals who are asked questions about how to perform a skill. The certified lab instructor (CLI) becomes a role model who must be a supportive coach for the students. New

York's lab instructor course is a 15-hour program that covers the essential instructional components needed for skill instruction.[26]

The New York system assures that assistant instructors have the instructional method training required. Not all states have this type of training program. As a primary instructor, plan meetings with the assistant instructors to teach the skills that are going to be taught. Making sure that the assistant instructors know what you want the students to learn is a step in the right direction.

The role of the assistant instructor cannot be underestimated. Successful programs are based upon the quality of their instruction. Good primary instruction is canceled out by ineffective assistant instructors' presentations. Choose the assistant instructors wisely. A lot is riding on who they are and what they do in a class. The assistant instructors are as important as any other component of the lesson plan. Prepare the assistant instructors with the same care that is put into designing the lesson plan. The end result may be an improved program and better assistant instructors.

Learning Phases

Students do not gain a mastery of a skill without proceeding through several steps on the way. Sometimes these steps are obvious, while other times they are merged together. Students tend to learn skills at different paces. This section looks at the different phases a student proceeds through to reach the mastery level.

Let's look at the four levels of skill learning:

1. Beginner (discovery)
2. Intermediate (plateau)
3. Advanced (latency)
4. Highly skilled (mastery)[27]

The parentheses identify alternate terms for each of the four levels. Either of the terms can be used when describing each level. To reach the highest level, a student must proceed in order from level 1 to level 4.

LEVEL 1: BEGINNER (DISCOVERY)

Students have to start somewhere, and it is at this level that they use the instructor's skill demonstration as their guideline to begin practice. Working with the assistant instructors, students start putting the skill together.

The students use a step-by-step approach to begin their learning process. Students tend to learn the skill rapidly in this phase. Errors are

---

[26]New York State EMS Certified Lab Instructor Curriculum, developed by the New York State Department of Health for the Training of Labs Skill Session Instructors (1988).
[27]Harrow, 1972.

made as they practice. At times, students look like they are all thumbs. This is when a caring and understanding coach is needed. This level is used to discover the correct methods for performing a skill. The learning is usually rapid in this phase. Helping the students put the skill together with improved speed and fewer errors sends the students on to the next level.

LEVEL 2: INTERMEDIATE (PLATEAU)

This is the second phase of learning. This phase can be very frustrating for students because the learning process is much slower. Students practice and practice but do not seem to have any more speed, accuracy, or form improvement. They are beginning to move from the step-by-step approach to a more integrated skill approach.

Also known as the plateau, students frequently repeat the same mistakes over and over. The instructor supervising the groups needs to stress the use of mental images. A video camera may help the students see their mistakes and correct them. A supportive coach will get the students out of this phase and on to the third level of learning.

LEVEL 3: ADVANCED (LATENCY)

At this level, students have usually progressed to indirect practice sessions. Students strive to improve their overall skill performance. Often, some students experience small errors that require an instructor's input and support. But for the majority of the students, a skill should be approaching the mastery level of performance.

The final touches for improving the speed and accuracy of the skill are practiced. As both of these improve, so does the form component. Instead of looking as if they have all thumbs, students are able to perform the skill with a fluid approach that begins to look like it is second nature. Adaptability is introduced by changing the situations, learning environments, or limiting the equipment for the skill. Once all the components are successfully demonstrated, the student enters the mastery level.

LEVEL 4: HIGHLY SKILLED (MASTERY LEVEL)

At the mastery level of performance, an Olympic athlete is expected to reach 9.95 to 10.0 scores. Likewise, emergency service personnel are expected to perform their duties at the mastery level of performance. But what exactly is the mastery level?

A student at the mastery level performs the skill with 100 percent confidence. The skill performance is secondary to other events happening around the student. The skill is performed flawlessly and with techniques that appear to be effortless. When confronted with a less than ideal setting, the student is able to adapt. The speed, accuracy, form, and adaptability components are at the level needed to perform the skill correctly.

In some training programs students may not reach this level of performance due to constraints on practice time, instructor reimbursement schedules, training facilities, and practice sessions, as well as peer pressure from seasoned personnel. An instructor attempts to control many of these factors, while others are not within the instructor's control. Still, victims trapped in a motor vehicle expect a 9.95 to 10.0 performance from the rescuers. It is up to an instructor to provide the training opportunities for students to attain the mastery level.

Postlogistics

Before a session ends, an instructor should begin to start the postlogistics. Often this means limiting the amount of practice time. Depending on the course, this may need to be a necessary trade-off. For example, a fire engine that is used in an all-day practice session will need complete servicing. Hoses need to be cleaned and restacked/replaced onto the hose bed; SCBA masks need to be serviced and any used SCBA bottles refilled; portable pumps and generators need to be serviced and cleaned; and the entire fire engine will need to be cleaned and restored to ready status. These tasks take time to complete. This is time that an instructor must incorporate into a skill practice session.

Returning an engine to ready status is a related skill activity. Students should not only be taught the proper use of emergency equipment but also how to restore the equipment to a ready status. In real life, there is no instructor to pick up the hose and reload it onto the truck. In a training program, an instructor should set up the equipment for the session. As for restoring the equipment after the session is over, this should be a class effort.

Summary

Instructing skill sessions requires a special instructor, one who is supportive and understanding.

Students tend to perform skills the way they are presented by their role model, the instructor. Initial referent contact is essential. Students need to see the whole demonstration before the specific parts of the skill are identified. The ideal speed, accuracy, and form of the skill must be presented to the students as the model to follow.

For students to reach the highly skilled (mastery) level of performance takes a lot of practice. This goal becomes both the students' and the instructor's objective for a skill session.

Assistant instructors play a vital role in the development of the students' skills. These assistants must mimic the lead instructor's educational traits. Principles related to performing a skill are stressed instead of specific methods. The assistant instructors are looked upon as being developmental coaches for the students. Students need to have honest information regarding their performance if they are to improve. Assistant instructors provide them with the good and weak aspects of a skill performance. Positive reinforcement of the aspects done correctly helps students repeat the skill correctly. Only caring and understanding coaches, ones who do not yell at the students, can accomplish this.

The mastery level is the highest level of performance. Quality care and performance begin with quality training. Factors that limit a student from attaining the mastery level should be addressed. Students need to be provided the opportunity to reach this goal.

Chapter 10
Evaluation Tools

➤ OBJECTIVES

- State the need to evaluate students.
- Identify the role of behavioral objectives.
- List types of evaluation tools.
- Identify types of evaluation tools:
  —Practical evaluations
  —Written evaluations
- Specify the composition, construction, delivery, and results of each assessment.
- Compare and contrast instructor-made examinations versus standardized examinations.
- Identify the role of test anxiety during evaluations.
- Identify the process for validating examinations.

EVALUATION KEYSTONE
Teachers have an obligation to provide their students with the best instruction possible. This implies that they must have some procedures whereby they can reliably and validly evaluate how effective their students have been taught.

William Mehrens and Irvin J. Lehmann[1]

The education process can be viewed as a jigsaw puzzle. You begin a puzzle with a box of pieces. You sort out the pieces and start to shape the outside border. Then piece by piece, the inside of the puzzle is assembled. Finally, there is one piece left, the "keystone piece." This piece finishes the puzzle and keeps the puzzle together. Only after the keystone piece is positioned is the puzzle complete.

The education process begins and ends with the behavioral objectives. The objectives are used to form the lesson plan. A lot of elements influence how students learn. To see if learning has occurred, some form of evaluation is used to see how many of the lesson plan's objectives have been met. The evaluation process helps the instructor determine if there has been a behavioral change, the "keystone piece." This chapter examines the types of evaluation tools that an instructor uses to assess the degree of learning achieved by the students.

---

[31]William J. Mehrens and Irvin J. Lehmann. *Measurement and Evaluation in Education and Psychology* (New York: Holt, Rinehart and Winston, 1978).

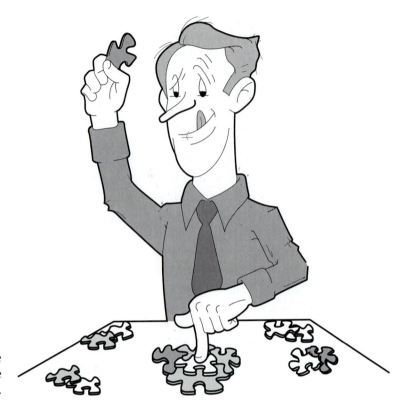

The keystone piece
keeps the puzzle
together.

Behavioral Objectives

Learning is invisible. Instructors become magicians to see if their students have learned the material. One could view an instructor as a magician, but the tricks of the trade that an instructor uses are not mystical. For a student to learn a subject, a change in behavior must occur. Instructors use various evaluation tools to assess if a behavioral change has occurred.

Well-written objectives help to predetermine the level of student performance that will be assessed. Let's look at the following objective:

The students will be able to select, correctly assemble, and use the power hydraulic spreader tool to safely remove a car door in less than 5 minutes.

This objective states the behavior that an instructor desires the students to accomplish. Objectives indirectly or directly help identify the type of evaluation tool to be used. An instructor uses various evaluation tools to measure the student's progress toward the lesson's objectives.

An instructor will use various evaluation tools throughout a course to see if learning is occurring. The following example shows how different evaluation tools can be used to evaluate a variety of learning abilities:

Knowledge   The instructor asks the following oral question.

Can someone list the organs associated with the digestive system?

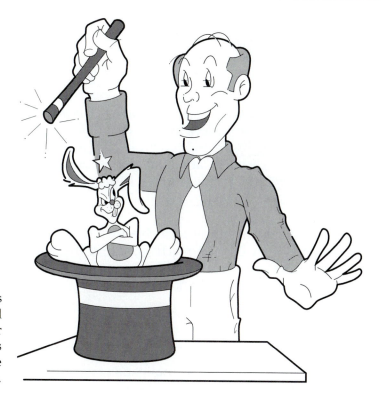

Poof . . . learning is invisible. Using well constructed behavior objectives makes learning become visible.

Comprehension   A written multiple-choice question.

> *Your engine is first in on a fully involved one-story house fire. You are the engineer. Which of the following is not your responsibility?*
> *A. Setting the pump in gear.*
> *B. Priming the pump.*
> *C. Grabbing the attack line and ladder.*
> *D. Establishing a water supply.*

Application   A practical evaluation scenario.

> *Your EMS crew has been dispatched to a high rise. Your patient is an elderly female lying at the bottom of a stairway. Outward rotation of the right leg is apparent. Patient complains of severe pain in the upper right leg and hip. No loss of consciousness.*

Analysis   An essay question.

> *There have been years of debate concerning high-pressure hoses versus high-volume hoses for direct fire suppression. Compare the two approaches and identify the positive and negative aspects of both approaches.*

Synthesis   An essay question.

> *You are the rescue captain at the scene of a motor vehicle accident. A car has plunged into a creek and all but the roof of the car is submerged. Victims are presumed trapped inside the car. You have the resources of*

a complete heavy rescue unit. What means of access and disentanglement would you choose?

Evaluation   An oral question.

You are dispatched to an isolated portion of your coverage area. A painting crew has been working on a 70-foot-high tension tower. One of the crew has become unconscious and is suspended by his ladder belt, which is clipped to the side of the tower. A rain storm is approaching with lightning and high winds. How would you effect a rescue in this situation?

The taxonomy of educational objectives (see Chapter 5) is used to help determine the evaluation mechanism and the difficulty of the evaluation. High-order tasks (analysis, synthesis, and evaluation) need to be mixed with the low-order tasks (knowledge, comprehension, and application).

Purpose of Evaluating

Aside from the instructor's obligation to incorporate some form of evaluation into the learning process, there are specific reasons for evaluating the learning process:

1. An evaluation measures a student's progress toward the behavioral objectives for the lesson.
2. The evaluation serves as a feedback mechanism for both the instructor and the students. The students and instructor can identify areas of weaknesses and strengths, for individual students as well as for the entire class.
3. The evaluation process can be used to measure the program, as well as the instructor's effectiveness. This should not be viewed as a sole indicator of instructor performance. It can be used to highlight positive and negative levels of performance that can be explored by other program evaluation mechanisms.
4. The evaluation is a learning experience. Further information on this topic is discussed in another part of this chapter.

For an instructor to assess the amount of learning, more than one type of evaluation tool is used. The evaluation process must assess both the knowledge and practical aspects of the learning process. Both these aspects need to be assessed before an instructor can say learning has taken place.

Evaluation Tools

Auto mechanics have a lot of tools in their toolbox. Instructors too have a lot of evaluation tools in their evaluation toolbox. An instructor uses evaluation tools to measure if a behavioral change has occurred.

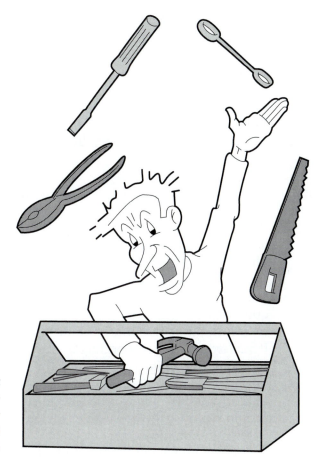

Instructors must select the right evaluation tool to determine if learning has occurred.

Oral Questions

In Chapter 8, the uses of oral questions were identified. Instructors use oral questions for a variety of purposes:

1. Stimulate discussions
2. Clarify points of concern
3. Review previously covered material
4. Evaluate the instructional effectiveness

Instructors can see if learning has occurred by the type of feedback they get from the students.

The four formats used to ask oral questions are recall, convergent, divergent, and value.[2]

Examples of the four formats are:

Knowledge or Recall: "What is the meaning of a placard that is red and has white lettering and blue bars?"

---

[2]Arthur A. Carm and Robert Sund. *Developing Questioning Techniques: A Self-Concept Approach* (New York: Merrill, 1971).

Convergent: "You are at a one-vehicle accident. The vehicle is a mid-size car. The victim is inside, and the driver's door is jammed against a tree. What means of access could you use to reach the victim?"
Divergent: "If a chlorine tanker truck wrecks in the middle of the downtown business district on a weekday and begins leaking, how would you respond?"
Value: "How would you feel about treating a patient with a disease that is fatal and could be contracted by being exposed to the patient's body fluids?"

Points to remember when asking oral questions:

- Prewrite oral questions into the lesson plan at the point of the lesson you intend to ask them.
- The questions meet the behavioral objectives.
- Challenge students to use their problem-solving abilities, but at the same time, do not overwhelm them with multiple questions.
- Allow the students sufficient time to respond to the questions. If students are not responding to a question, and it is a recall level question, this may be telling the instructor that learning may not be taking place. For problem-solving questions, an instructor, after giving sufficient time to answer the question, should rephrase the question or review the material relating to the question.
- Positive reinforcement of the student answers. Even a student's wrong answer can have positive reinforcement. An example would be, "No, that's not the exact answer that I was looking for. . . ."
- Avoid picking on any one student. Share the questions with all the students. Students may begin to rely upon one or two students answering the questions.

Oral questions are a powerful evaluation tool. Instructors who can mix question formats into the flow of their lesson presentation can accomplish learning and evaluation at the same time. Oral questions are only one evaluation tool. Look at both written and practical forms of evaluation before deciding upon a student's true knowledge of the material.

Practical Evaluations

To perform a skill requires students to harmonize their cognitive, psychomotor abilities, and affective domains. All three educational domains influence a student's ability to perform a skill. Chapter 9 looked at how students learn and practice skills. Instructors tend to nurture a student's skill development throughout a training program. Periodically throughout a program there should be an assessment of a student's skill proficiency. How, who, and what to assess are discussed in this section (Figure 10-1).

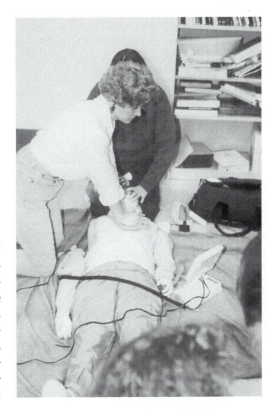

Figure 10-1
To perform a practical skill, a student requires knowledge (cognitive domain), skill practice (psychomotor domain), and effective communication skills (affective domain).

PRACTICAL EVALUATION TOOLS

There are two practical tools used to assess skills:

1. End-product evaluation
2. Process evaluation[3]

The end-product practical evaluation focuses on a student's ability to problem-solve situations. Instructors (i.e., evaluators) review the final outcome and compliance with a skill's critical performance criteria. Critical performance criteria specify performance steps necessary for correct performance of a skill. A student's ability to use creativity, resourcefulness, and inventiveness influences whether a skill is performed correctly.

The process evaluation is a step-by-step evaluation. Using the task analysis, a skill is dissected into its component parts. The instructor assesses the student's ability to complete steps 1, 2, 3, 4, and so on in a specific order.

If an instructor has just completed the initial instruction of a skill, such as the application of the hare traction splint, the process evaluation would be appropriate to use. An instructor would want to identify inaccurate methods of the splint's application. As the course progresses, students should be integrating multiple skills. The end-product approach would be

---

[3]Mehrens and Lehmann, 1978.

the preferred evaluation tool in assessing the "whole treatment" of a patient. The final outcome and critical performance criteria, not the specific sequential steps used to accomplish the skill, are assessed. The end-product evaluation is closer to real life situations than the process approach. Both approaches have their place during a training program. How to use these approaches is discussed in the next section.

DESIGNING THE PRACTICAL EXAMINATION

An instructor faces unique logistical challenges when designing a practical exam. Some of the decisions facing an instructor include the development of testing scenarios, identification of critical performance criteria, determining the number of practical stations, identifying the equipment needed for the exam, identifying and selecting instructors to be station evaluators, a safety officer when appropriate, and designing the evaluation scoring sheets.

A testing scenario defines the performance expectations for the students. Items included in a scenario are:

- Lesson or section name
- Makeup/moulage/props
- Number of victims
- Station equipment
- Victim programming
- The scenario
- Supplemental scenario information (a patient's vital signs, hose pressure, scene safety, etc.)
- Number of station evaluators
- Expected performance objectives
- Scoring criteria

Number of Stations
How many stations are needed? How many psychomotor objectives were covered in the lesson? What is important for the students to know and use in the field? To answer these questions, the following criteria can assist an instructor in determining the number of testing stations.

- Identify the number and types of behavioral objectives that are skill oriented.
- Decide on what skills can be evaluated by which evaluation tool.
- Time is a key factor. Consideration must be given to the time that it will take for the students to complete a station. For example, if you are testing a group of students in CPR and airway adjuncts, it is possible to evaluate them in less than 10 minutes. Conversely a rescue scenario may take 45 minutes to complete.
- Equipment and resources may place restrictions on the number of stations. Victims, wrecked autos, burn building, training equipment, moulage person, and a host of other resources affect the number and type of stations.

- Availability of evaluators for the exam. Third-party evaluators should be the preferred choice. Attaining evaluators for the session may determine how many stations to schedule.
- Well-written examination scenarios take time to construct. Not all instructors have a lot of extra time to create complex scenarios.

After reviewing these determinants, place them into a priority format. Identify those skill stations that can be accomplished in the time allotted for the class session, given the available resources.

Realism

To make a situation appear real requires the use of realism concepts (Figure 10-2). Chapter 13 identifies realism concepts used to enhance and create realistic situations. During a practical evaluation, the use of realism becomes paramount. Every attempt should be made to include realism into each phase of the evaluation process.

Appropriate makeup of the victims enhances the visual perceptions of the student. Appropriate acting by a patient actor is required. Smoke, fire, wrecked vehicles, dim lighting, and burned clothing can be used to add realism to a scenario.

Equipment

The type of equipment used for the examination should be the type of equipment used throughout the program. If students trained on a 1,500-gallon-per-minute (gpm) pumper, it would be inappropriate to examine them on a 500-gpm pumper, especially if it is a different make and style.

Adequate equipment for the station becomes a factor. To have students pretend equipment exists defeats the purpose of the evaluation. Lay out the equipment at the stations before the examination. Use a checklist to assure that there is enough equipment for the stations. Have spare pieces of equipment on hand. During an examination, a piece of equipment may break and need to be replaced.

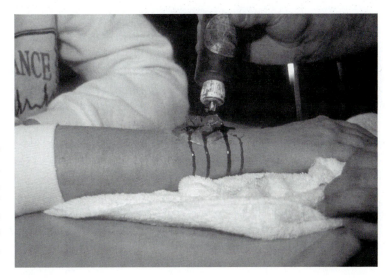

Figure 10-2
Makeup and moulage are realism components not only for classroom use but also for use during practical examinations.

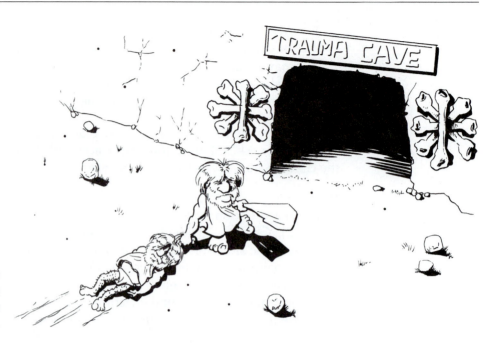

Instructors need to prevent accidents and not be the cause of them.

The instructor should assure that the equipment for the stations is in working order. All equipment is known to break down at the worst possible moment. Testing the equipment before the examination can minimize equipment breakdowns during the examination. This includes checking fluid levels in engines, air supply in air bottles, and electric supply in battery-operated equipment. Instructors need to see the students using the equipment, not pretending to use it.

STUDENT BRIEFING

An instructor must orient students about the examination. A student's anxiety level for an examination can be lessened by a calm and reassuring description of the evaluation process. Students need to know what is going to be expected of them during the evaluation. Items to include are:

1. Number of stations for the examination
2. Student rotation between the testing stations
3. Overview of the examination objectives for each station (e.g., at the hose laying station you will be expected to lay the appropriate hose type and provide water supply to the engine)
4. Grading criteria being used during the examination
5. Retest options for the examination
6. Debriefing area to disclose examination scores

EVALUATORS

An instructor needs to select and use evaluators who will provide an honest review of the students. Ideally the evaluators should not have any ties to the class, professionally or personally. An instructor often cannot assure this. These factors can influence the validity of the examination.

During a practical examination, an evaluator's attitude and action can contribute to an inaccurate assessment of the students. There are evaluator errors that the lead instructor should monitor during a practical evaluation. Those errors are:

1. *Halo effect:* An evaluator's personal attitude toward a student being tested influences the station's score. This could be either a positive or negative score. To lessen this error, an evaluator who does not know the student should test the student.

2. *Teaching at the station:* Evaluators often face an overwhelming desire to jump into the examination and correct a student's mistakes. If this happens, invalid scores for the station result. The purpose of the evaluation is to identify the positive and weak aspects of the learning experience. An evaluator should refrain from interrupting the students during the examination.

3. *Generosity/leniency error:* Some evaluators feel uneasy assigning weak or poor scores to students. "In a real setting they wouldn't do that," or "They had the basic concept, it wasn't really that bad." When an evaluator makes these types of comments, a red flag should go up. The lead instructor should closely review that evaluator's findings. Evaluators demonstrating these characteristics will commonly overrate the performance of the students. This directly reduces the validity and increases the error rate of the evaluation. Using critical performance criteria helps to reduce this error.

4. *Central tendency error:* The evaluator chooses the middle of the road for all the students they evaluate. There is little flexibility in one direction or the other. Average scores, average performance comments, and no super performance or terrible comments are identified. Clearly written skill check sheets may help lessen this error tendency.[4]

Instructors should try to use evaluators who have completed an evaluator training course. Evaluations depend upon the evaluator's ability to observe, accurately recall, and interpret the information. Evaluators who try to remember the student's performance will inaccurately record the information 25 percent of the time. One educational account suggests that an evaluator become "machinelike" when evaluating, recording only the facts, not the evaluator's subjective viewpoints. Evaluating in this manner will lead to a valid examination and a performance score that is easily defended.[5]

Instructors tend to use evaluators who consistently provide honest evaluations. These evaluators provide both positive and negative feedback, use objective-based skill criteria, and desire quality-trained individuals from the training program. These evaluators recognize when students are excessively nervous and attempt to calm them down, and they allow the students an opportunity to perform the skill.

---

[4]From *Principles of Educational and Psychological Measurement and Evaluation, 3rd edition,* by G. Sax © 1989. Reprinted with permission of Wadsworth, an imprint of the Wadsworth Group, a division of Thomson Learning. Fax 800 730-2215.
[5]Ibid.

CHECKLISTS AND CRITICAL SCORING CRITERIA

The checklist enables the evaluator to observe and record specific behaviors (skills), performed by the student. A well-prepared checklist provides:

1. The evaluator with specific behaviors to observe during the skill
2. An easy mechanism for recording student performance

An end-product checklist contains broad objectives and critical performance criteria. The objectives focus on the completion of the entire situation. The process checklist identifies a skill's specific steps. Students are rated upon the completion of the skill's steps in a specific sequence. If the students do not complete the steps in the correct order, an unsatisfactory score is indicated. A numeric or letter scoring system is used for either checklist. Items to include in a checklist are:

1. Title
2. Student name(s)
3. Time begun and time ended
4. Grading criteria
5. Documentation section
6. Evaluator name(s)

SCORING OF STUDENTS

You have failed the examination! No retest opportunity!

These phrases can be devastating to a student. The purpose of an evaluation is to measure a student's ability and identify how to improve their performance. Terms such as *satisfactory* or *unsatisfactory* are often used as grade indicators. An unsatisfactory score means that certain skill components were not performed correctly. This differs from *failure*, which denotes finality and no chance for improvement. If a student attains an unsatisfactory score, the student must be made aware of the error or errors. Full knowledge of the results is a key aspect of learning a skill[6] (see Chapter 9).

The Written Examination

Written examinations have been placed onto a false pedestal where there is no other reliable form of examination. Many of the least reliable exams are written exams. A variety of evaluation tools are used to see if students are learning. These tools include oral, practical, experiential, value, and of course written examinations.

---

[6]Robert N. Singer. *Motor Learning and Human Performance*, 3rd ed. (New York: Macmillan, 1980).

The written examination is the most common and widely used evaluation tool. From business owners to the lay public, the benchmark of whether students are considered competent rests upon whether or not they passed the written examination. "If you passed the written exam you must know what you're doing" is a commonly heard phrase. These types of comments and attitudes can be, and often are, false impressions of a student's learning abilities. Review the section dealing with learning styles in Chapter 2. Not everyone is a book-smart learner, and many students do not perform well on written exams. There are countless variables as to why a student performed in the manner that was observed. For example, students who are psychomotor oriented in their daily jobs will likely do well on a practical examination, as well as on oral examinations. Conversely, these same students may do terribly on the written examination, in part, due to the lack of written stimulation in their daily lives. These students, without intense instructor support, will not have high scores on the written examination. Instructors need to identify these students, show them how to study the lesson material, and how to take written examinations.

Additional factors influencing test scores include student illness, test anxiety, poorly written test items, too much noise in the testing area, an incorrect answer key, an invalid examination, lack of student preparation, poor instruction, or poor course materials. These and other factors may effect a student's performance on the written examination, or for that matter, for any form of evaluation.

OBJECTIVITY AND SUBJECTIVITY

Regardless of the type of evaluation tool that is being used, an examination must be an objective assessment. The word *objective* means to be without bias or prejudice toward another; impersonal. When designing examinations, instructors need to make them as objective as possible. Depending on the type of examination, there is always a degree of subjectivity.

Subjectivity occurs when instructors' attitudes, opinions, or values influence their judgment of a student's performance. Subjectivity also occurs when an examination cannot be referenced by an external source. Practical and value-based assessments are inherently subjective. Subjectivity cannot be totally erased when using some examination formats (i.e., essay or practical evaluations) but it can be minimized. In a previous section dealing with evaluators, ways to minimize evaluator bias were discussed. In successive sections, various written examinations will be discussed. The degrees of objectivity and subjectivity with each type of examination will be identified.

PLANNING THE WRITTEN EXAMINATION: "THE TEST BLUEPRINT"

Building contractors use blueprints to construct houses and buildings. The plumbing, electrical wiring, fixtures, fireplace, and so on are identified. Without a blueprint to follow, construction workers would be lost. The blueprint defines the entire construction process in precise detail. The same principle holds true for instructors. Instructors need to have a blueprint to follow when developing and using evaluation tools. A test blueprint is especially needed for written examinations.

Test blueprints are based on a lesson's objectives and/or the time spent covering the lesson material. The construction of a blueprint is directly based upon the number of examination questions: 25, 50, 75, 100, and so on. A percentage is calculated for each determinant. A formula for determining the number of examination questions looks like this:

Total exam questions $\times$ % of objectives = No. specific questions[7]

Use the same formula for calculating the amount of classroom time spent on the subject.

An instructor compares the percentages and selects the percentage that best reflects the emphasis and importance of the subject material that was covered during the course. Figure 10-3 shows the relationship of the lesson objectives, class time spent, and the taxonomy of educational objectives for the creation of the blueprint.

The decision for the number of examination questions is arbitrary. Time, the type of examination being used, and the amount of material covered are all factors that must be considered. For example, a student should be given at least 1 minute for each multiple-choice question. A fifty-question examination should have a time limit of 50 minutes to 1 hour. The instructor needs to have enough questions to ensure adequate coverage of the material covered during the lesson.

ESSAY

The essay examination is a powerful evaluation tool used in the right setting. An instructor needs to be aware of the performance levels of the students before deciding upon the essay examination. The essay examination is not for every group of students.

Essay examinations can provide students with the ability to express creative thinking. The essay examination works extremely well for evaluating small groups of students. Instructors also benefit from the short preparation time to create the examination, as compared to the lengthy time it takes to write a multiple-choice examination.

There are limitations associated with the essay examination. A critical limitation is the subjectivity. Opinions or attitudes regarding a student can influence the instructor, and thus the student's score. Other factors associated with the essay include:

1. It is difficult to score an essay question objectively.
2. Limited aspects of the student's knowledge are being assessed. Instead of many objectives being reviewed, only specific lesson objectives are evaluated.

---

[7]Janet A. Head. *Instructor Resource Manual* (Upper Saddle River, N.J.: Prentice Hall, 1990).

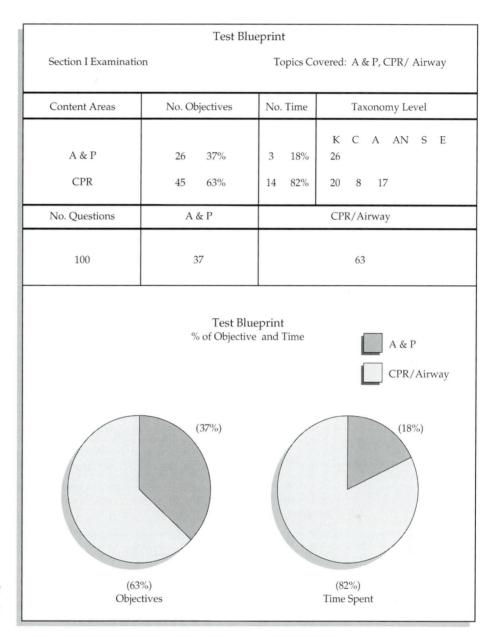

Test Blueprint			
Section I Examination			Topics Covered: A & P, CPR/ Airway

Content Areas	No. Objectives	No. Time	Taxonomy Level
			K C A AN S E
A & P	26 37%	3 18%	26
CPR	45 63%	14 82%	20 8 17

No. Questions	A & P	CPR/Airway
100	37	63

Test Blueprint
% of Objective and Time

A & P

CPR/Airway

(37%)

(18%)

(63%)
Objectives

(82%)
Time Spent

Figure 10-3
Sample test
blueprint.

3. The essay examination is time consuming for both the instructor and the student. Essays take up valuable classroom time. Students have to manually write out the answers to a question. It can take hours of nonclassroom time for the instructor to correct the examinations.

4. Essay examinations can encourage student memorization of the material. Facts are studied for the short-term learning and the actual concepts are not learned by the students.

5. Students may not completely understand the meaning of the essay question. Thus, the student's answer may not even be close to the answer that the instructor is looking for.

6. Other factors, grammar, spelling, and writing style, are often evaluated with the overall content that is being assessed.

Writing the Essay Examination

First, an instructor must decide which objectives are the most important for the students to know. Only these objectives will be covered in an essay test. Not being able to test multiple behavioral objectives limits the use of the essay test in many courses.

The time allotted for the examination becomes a factor in how the exam is developed. For example, if there is one hour of classroom time for an examination, then the essay exam should consist of two or three short questions.

How are essay questions written? The following are issues to consider when writing an essay question:

1. State the specific content of the information being asked. For example, a question asks, "Identify the operation of a fire extinguisher." This question can be interpreted in many ways. Is it a dry chemical extinguisher or an AFFF water extinguisher? Another way of writing this question is, "Describe the procedure for using an AFFF water extinguisher on an oil fire."
2. Use descriptive words: *define, outline, select,* and *compare/contrast.* These terms provide a student with a working idea of the answer that is being sought.
3. Limit the scope of the student's answers. Clearly state the length of the answer. This gives the student a framework for responding to the question. On the examination form, limiting the space to write the answer can be a helpful tool to define a student's response.
4. Allow sufficient time for the students to respond to each question. Short-answer responses, those around half a page, take students around 10 to 15 minutes to answer. Full-page responses can take 20 to 30 minutes to answer.
5. Write the "perfect" answer to each question. Reference the objective that the question is based on. Prewritten answers will improve an examination's validity.[8]

Correcting the Essay Examination

The key to correcting the essay examination is to limit subjectivity. Methods that can be used are:

1. Use a correct answer key that was made when the examination was developed. Compare each of the student's answers to the key words and concepts contained within the answer key.
2. When correcting the examinations, place a sheet of paper over the student's name. Although the handwriting of the student can still be recognized, in many cases, hiding the name helps reduce the halo effect.
3. Use a third-party instructor to correct the examinations. Ideally, this is an instructor who does not know any of the students. They are provided the answer key and the student's answer sheets.

---

[8]Mehrens and Lehmann, 1978.

4. To assist a third-party instructor, the creation of a scoring system is often useful. Identifying key words will permit easy correction of the examinations.

5. Whoever grades the examinations, grade only one question at a time for all the examinations. This promotes an equal grading pattern for the answers to the questions on all the examinations.

6. Provide written comments on the student's answer sheets. Clearly identify the correct answer. Denote the student's score as it compares to the total possible score.[9,10]

Correcting essay examinations can be a challenging proposition for an instructor. Assuring that the subjectivity of the grades is kept to a minimum is not easy. It takes a lot of time to grade essay examinations. Be sure to allow

Exhibit 10-1

Essay Examination

NAME: _____

COURSE TITLE: _____

DIRECTIONS: Read each question fully before writing the answer. Use the allotted space to respond to the question. You will have 1 hour to complete the examination. Return your examination to the monitor when completed. DO NOT BEGIN UNTIL TOLD TO START!

1. You are dispatched to the scene of a two-vehicle MVA. The vehicles are wrecked in a head-on type collision. Both drivers are trapped inside the vehicles. Identify the main concerns you have as the crew chief of the responding unit.

_____
_____
_____
_____
_____

2. Describe and list situations at the scene of an MVA that would make it necessary for all personnel to wear an SCBA.

_____
_____
_____
_____
_____

---

[9]Sax, 1989.
[10]Mehrens and Lehmann, 1978.

sufficient time to correct the examination. Exhibit 10-1 is an example of an essay examination that could be used in an emergency service classroom.

(Insert the CD Rom. Click on the examination development file folder. Click on the index or setup icon. The program reviews types of examinations.)

SHORT-ANSWER AND COMPLETION QUESTIONS

Short-answer and completion examinations are mainly used for quizzes or small-unit examinations. There are differences between the two examination formats. The completion examination consists of one- or two-word answers. Short-answer examinations usually require a student to write one or two sentences to answer the question.

Advantages to these exams include:

- Both of the examinations are easily written.
- The guessing factor is less compared to other exams.
- There can be an increased number of test items, and this format is more objective than is the essay exam.

There are also disadvantages to these exams.

1. At the top of the list is subjectivity. Unless the "correct" answers are written down prior to the examination, subjectivity becomes a factor.
2. Memorizing the information, versus knowing the information, commonly occurs when using this format.
3. Some instructors find difficulty physically correcting these examinations. This is often linked to the format of the examination. A well-written format reduces this problem.

MATCHING EXAMINATION

The test blueprint determines whether the examination should be used. An instructor needs to identify the objectives and terms that lend themselves to an association–based format.

The matching format contains two separate columns. One column contains the question or statement. It is then matched to a list of potential answers in a second column. Depending on how a matching exam is set up, answers can be used several times or only once. There are always more answers than questions. The distracter answers must be close to the correct answer to cause a choice between the answers.

The examination directions must specify the examination's format. For example, can an answer be used more than once? What does each column mean? Where is the student's answer written? The matching exam directions must specify the actions that students are to make when answering a matching question.

TRUE-AND-FALSE EXAMINATION

When an instructor has a lot of factual material to review, a true-and-false (T/F) examination should be considered. A lot of test items can be assessed in a very short time using the T/F format.

In the T/F examination there are only two possible answers. This presents the biggest downfall of the T/F examination, the guessing factor. An instructor cannot be sure if students know the material or whether they guessed the answer. It is a fifty-fifty chance, with those being the minimum odds. If questions are incorrectly phrased, the guessing factor increases.

Another pitfall of the T/F examination is the memorization of the lesson material. Instead of gaining an understanding of the material, students cram their short-term memories with factual information, which unless it is reinforced will be forgotten soon after the exam.

Students who know how to take a T/F exam can improve their guessing by knowing certain key words. Table 10-1 lists words that tend to be true or false.[11]

CONSIDERATIONS FOR OBJECTIVE EXAMINATIONS

When designing a short-answer, matching, true/false, or even a multiple-choice examination, an instructor should consider these elements:

1. Identify the knowledge and information that are important to know. Some instructors often test trivial information. This tends to cause students to be frustrated and results in inaccurate information.
2. Design the examination around the students. The student's age, ability level, and the rationale for giving the examination become important determinants. For example, using "thousand-dollar words" with a group of individuals who have learning disabilities would be inappropriate.

Table 10-1 Key Words in True-and-False Examinations

True Key Words	False Key Words
should	only
may	alone
most	all
some	none
often	always
generally	never

---

[11]Ibid.

3. Write the questions to a specific point. Avoid excessive language. Use only as many words as are necessary. Remember, keep the terms and phrases to the level of the students.
4. Do not use direct quotes from the textbook, such as leaving a key word out and inserting a blank line. The meaning of the statement is easily lost when using this technique.
5. Do not write questions that are related so that one question's answer makes the rest of the answers incorrect.
6. Avoid providing the answer to another question in a different section of the examination.
7. Design the question and possible answers so that there is only one "best" or correct answer to the question.
8. Avoid inserting a negative word or phrase into a positive statement to make it incorrect.
9. When formatting the examination, do not have questions or answers run over onto the next page. This is especially important for matching and multiple-choice questions. The selection of the answers or the stem to the question being on a different page creates unnecessary reading difficulty for the student. When formatting the questions, flip the ordering of the questions around to fit them into the examination format.

MULTIPLE-CHOICE EXAMINATION

To many instructors, there is no other examination, there is only the multiple-choice examination. By far, the multiple-choice examination is the most popular examination. The multiple uses and options associated with this format make it the most widely used examination.[12] Although the most popular examination, it is also the most challenging examination for an instructor to write.

The basic format consists of two parts, a stem and a set of answers. The stem can be a sentence, problem, paragraph, or a diagram. The answers consist of four, five, or six different choices, with only *one* correct answer among the choices. The key is to have the incorrect answers, known as distracters, be totally incorrect but believable.

Multiple-choice examination formats are

1. Multiple response
2. Best answer
3. Sentence completion
4. Question
5. Interpretative

Writing the Multiple-Choice Question
The following are general principles used to create the multiple-choice question and answers.

---

[12]Ibid.

1. The stem is to be a written statement that clearly identifies background information as well as the question. If the question is well written, a student should have a working idea of the answer without even looking at the possible answers.

2. Use penny terms and avoid ten-dollar terms. If terms are key learning objectives, then test them. It is not appropriate to "jazz up" the exam by using complex terms that are not used in everyday settings.

3. The stem should be a complete sentence or statement. Avoid incomplete sentences or questions.

4. The distracters must be related to the subject being evaluated. However, the distracters must be 100 percent incorrect.[13] This presents a unique situation; how can an answer be close but still be incorrect? Let's look at the following example from a rescue examination. *A* is the correct answer.

   Of the following equipment, which item(s) is/are used for gaining access into a wrecked vehicle?
   1. Center punch
   2. 4 × 4 cribbing
   3. Pry bar
   4. Power hydraulic spreader tool

   A. 1 only
   B. 2, 4 only
   C. 3 only
   D. 1, 3, 4 only

5. The correct answer should be the same length as the distracters. Often students can guess the right answer by looking at the longest answer. There can be only one correct answer.

6. "Watch your grammar!" No, this is not your high school English teacher talking, but then again maybe it is. Plurals and singular terms in the stem can establish the type of answer for the question. The alternatives listed below the question need to match the grammar of the stem. As seen above in principle 4, giving a choice of either a plural or singular alternative in the stem allows the distracters and answers to coincide.

7. "All of the above" or "None of the above" are distracters that should be limited in their use. Identify "real" distracters and avoid these options whenever possible.

8. There are no specific numbers of distracters. Most instructors use four- five- or six-answer sets. There appears to be no significant difference in the reliability of a four-answer format versus a six-answer format.[14] If you are using computer-graded answer sheets, check the number of possible answer spaces. Most computer answer sheets allow up to six-answer sets.

---

[13]Sax, 1989.
[14]Mehrens and Lehmann, 1978.

9. When writing the questions and distracters, be sure not to provide answers to other questions on the examination. Students will look back at previously answered questions to attain answers to other questions on the examination.

10. "All stems are not created equal!" Based upon the material being covered, the stem could consist of a photograph, drawing, map, ECG strip, or a short case-study paragraph. Below each of these formats, a one-, two-, or three-question/answer set can be constructed. This style of question is associated with the interpretation format.

11. Balance the correct answers. If an examination is to be 100 questions in length with four-answer selections, ideally there should be 25 *A*, 25 *B*, 25 *C*, and 25 *D* answers. Often students will follow a guessing approach of, "If I do not know the answer I'll pick answer *C*." A balanced examination eliminates the guessing option.

12. The answer selections should appear below the stem. If possible, the answers should be indented five spaces from the left margin. This offsets the answers from the stem and makes the answers stick out from the stem.

13. Key words in the stem should be highlighted. These key words are words that are not common to the majority of the other questions. Words like ALL, **NOT,** <u>except for,</u> or *best* can be highlighted in various ways. These words are highlighted to show the student a unique situation or viewpoint.

14. Answers and questions must stay on the same page. Multiple-choice questions take up a lot of space. Questions and answers that run over onto an adjacent page cause an unnecessary interruption in a student's train of thought. This is especially true when students have to flip the page over and over to read all the answers.

15. Answer formats for the examination need to be consistent. For example, if the answers are positioned in the following manner:

    A.   A.   C.
    B.   or   B.   D.
    C.
    D.

    Keep the same format throughout the examination. Do not mix the ordering of the examination answer format. It causes unnecessary confusion and may cause the student to answer the question incorrectly.

16. The time of the examination needs to be identified. Each multiple-choice question should have 1 minute set aside. This will mean that a fifty-question examination will take 50 minutes to complete.[15]

---

[15]Pennsylvania Department of Health. *Examination Study Guide and Instructor Curriculum* (Harrisburg, Penn.: 1989).

Designing good multiple-choice questions is not an easy task. Instructors must set aside sufficient time to create the examinations. Each exam should fairly and accurately evaluate the student's learning growth. Evaluating students with an objective evaluation tool allows the instructor to closely monitor the learning growth of the students. The multiple-choice examination provides the avenue for an objective review of the students, which is a key goal when using any evaluation tool.

EXAMINATION DIRECTIONS

A common thread among all the written examinations, as well as for the practical examination, is to have well-written directions. Knowing what is expected by the instructor helps the students during the examination. Directions should include:

- Advising the student to read the whole question before answering the question. This would include the stem, a short paragraph, and all the potential answers.
- Method of documentation. Are the answers written onto the booklet, onto a separate answer sheet, or onto a computer answer sheet or entered directly into the computer?
- Examination booklets. If an examination booklet is being used, stress the need not to make any stray marks inside the booklet. Some instructors have found it useful to give a piece of scratch paper to all the students, so students can mark those questions that require additional thought.

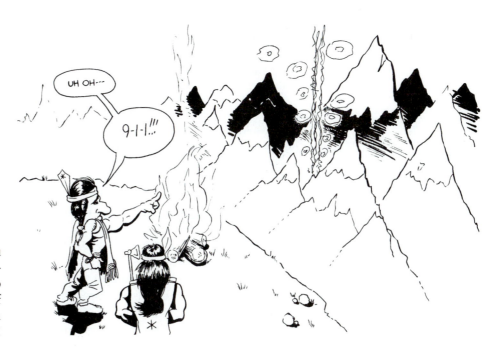

Make sure you clearly state exam directions. You need to know what kind of smoke signal you have sent up!

- Time. Specify the time allowed for the examination. This, combined with a stating of the time, allows the student to budget time for the examination.
- Instructor assistance during the examination. Often students have questions or concerns during the examination. A statement from the instructor regarding what questions and concerns will be addressed during the examination is appropriate. A blurred question, misspelled words, or a missing page are appropriate student concerns. Asking what the term *dyspnea* means would not be an appropriate question that an instructor should respond to.
- Starting the examination. Identify the specific procedures that you want followed for starting the examination. Many students wish to get a head start on the examination. Comments such as, "Start the examination only when instructed" or "You may start when you receive the examination booklet" are helpful.
- Ending the examination. When students complete the examination, are they to sit quietly in the room until everyone finishes; how do they hand in their examinations; can they go into an area outside the room after the examination; or are they permitted to go home after the examination? Any one of these options needs to be identified to the students. The written directions are the place to do just that.

THE ANSWER SHEET

Associated mainly with the multiple-choice examination, but used with any written evaluation tool, is the answer sheet. Written examination questions are not easily written, especially good multiple-choice questions. Separate answer sheets allow instructors to use examinations multiple times, at the same time reducing reproduction costs for the examination.

The answer sheet format can be a numbered sheet of paper with single lines beside each number. Example:

1. __

Some instructors type letters in a row, so that the student needs only to circle the answer. Example:

1. A B C D

One of the most popular answer sheet formats is the computer answer sheet. These answer sheets are designed for an "optiscanner" computer system (Figure 10-4). They consist of either lettered circles or lines, which are colored in with a pencil or pen. Instructors who do not have access to a computer entry system use these forms. An answer key is manually punched out for each correct answer. The instructor then places the answer key over a student's answer sheet and marks the incorrect responses.

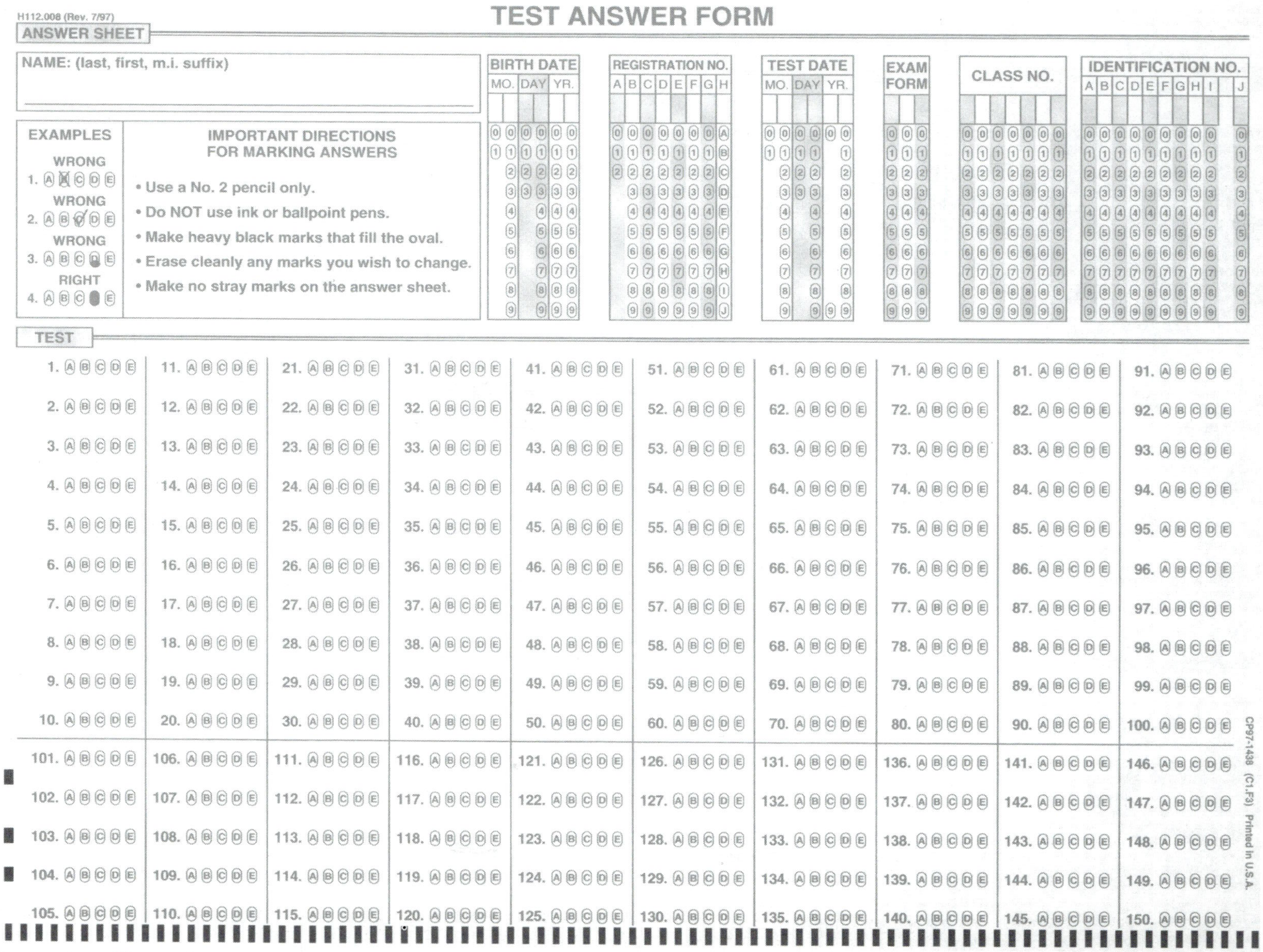
H112.008 (Rev. 7/97)

ANSWER SHEET

TEST ANSWER FORM

NAME: (last, first, m.i. suffix)

BIRTH DATE: MO. DAY YR.

REGISTRATION NO.: A B C D E F G H

TEST DATE: MO. DAY YR.

EXAM FORM

CLASS NO.

IDENTIFICATION NO.: A B C D E F G H I J

EXAMPLES

WRONG
1. A B C D E

WRONG
2. A B C D E

WRONG
3. A B C D E

RIGHT
4. A B C D E

IMPORTANT DIRECTIONS FOR MARKING ANSWERS

- Use a No. 2 pencil only.
- Do NOT use ink or ballpoint pens.
- Make heavy black marks that fill the oval.
- Erase cleanly any marks you wish to change.
- Make no stray marks on the answer sheet.

TEST

1. A B C D E	11. A B C D E	21. A B C D E	31. A B C D E	41. A B C D E	51. A B C D E	61. A B C D E	71. A B C D E	81. A B C D E	91. A B C D E
2. A B C D E	12. A B C D E	22. A B C D E	32. A B C D E	42. A B C D E	52. A B C D E	62. A B C D E	72. A B C D E	82. A B C D E	92. A B C D E
3. A B C D E	13. A B C D E	23. A B C D E	33. A B C D E	43. A B C D E	53. A B C D E	63. A B C D E	73. A B C D E	83. A B C D E	93. A B C D E
4. A B C D E	14. A B C D E	24. A B C D E	34. A B C D E	44. A B C D E	54. A B C D E	64. A B C D E	74. A B C D E	84. A B C D E	94. A B C D E
5. A B C D E	15. A B C D E	25. A B C D E	35. A B C D E	45. A B C D E	55. A B C D E	65. A B C D E	75. A B C D E	85. A B C D E	95. A B C D E
6. A B C D E	16. A B C D E	26. A B C D E	36. A B C D E	46. A B C D E	56. A B C D E	66. A B C D E	76. A B C D E	86. A B C D E	96. A B C D E
7. A B C D E	17. A B C D E	27. A B C D E	37. A B C D E	47. A B C D E	57. A B C D E	67. A B C D E	77. A B C D E	87. A B C D E	97. A B C D E
8. A B C D E	18. A B C D E	28. A B C D E	38. A B C D E	48. A B C D E	58. A B C D E	68. A B C D E	78. A B C D E	88. A B C D E	98. A B C D E
9. A B C D E	19. A B C D E	29. A B C D E	39. A B C D E	49. A B C D E	59. A B C D E	69. A B C D E	79. A B C D E	89. A B C D E	99. A B C D E
10. A B C D E	20. A B C D E	30. A B C D E	40. A B C D E	50. A B C D E	60. A B C D E	70. A B C D E	80. A B C D E	90. A B C D E	100. A B C D E
101. A B C D E	106. A B C D E	111. A B C D E	116. A B C D E	121. A B C D E	126. A B C D E	131. A B C D E	136. A B C D E	141. A B C D E	146. A B C D E
102. A B C D E	107. A B C D E	112. A B C D E	117. A B C D E	122. A B C D E	127. A B C D E	132. A B C D E	137. A B C D E	142. A B C D E	147. A B C D E
103. A B C D E	108. A B C D E	113. A B C D E	118. A B C D E	123. A B C D E	128. A B C D E	133. A B C D E	138. A B C D E	143. A B C D E	148. A B C D E
104. A B C D E	109. A B C D E	114. A B C D E	119. A B C D E	124. A B C D E	129. A B C D E	134. A B C D E	139. A B C D E	144. A B C D E	149. A B C D E
105. A B C D E	110. A B C D E	115. A B C D E	120. A B C D E	125. A B C D E	130. A B C D E	135. A B C D E	140. A B C D E	145. A B C D E	150. A B C D E

CP97-1438 (C1.F3) Printed in U.S.A.

Figure 10-4 Photo of an optiscan form.

Benefits to using answer sheets are:

- Easy correction by the instructor.
- Multiple use of examinations.
- Standard recording format.
- Computer-coded sheets can prepare students for standardized examination formats.
- Computer-entered examinations are quickly graded and an examination analysis can be easily created.
- Reduced reproduction costs for the examination.

Teacher-Made Examinations Versus Standardized Tests

Through all aspects of education, a lengthy debate has been going on for years concerning the use of standardized examinations versus teacher-made examinations. Both sides of the issue have noteworthy perspectives. Those on the teacher-made side maintain that they know their students' educational strengths and weaknesses. They feel that they can design the examination to meet the learning capabilities of their students. A teacher-made examination measures the educational growth for a specific group of students. The standardized examination perspective maintains that a standardized examination will provide a better objective review of the student's learning growth. The standardized examination can provide a state or national form of measurement.

There are commercially made examinations available for EMS and fire training programs. These examinations are keyed to the student's textbooks. There are also computer test banks that are keyed to specific curriculum material. These are "semistandardized" examinations. The actual instructor does not make the questions. A professional educator makes them for use across the nation. This nationwide distribution allows these examinations to fall into the standardized examination category.

There are nationally accredited examinations. In EMS, there is the National Registry of EMTs examination. EMT-B, EMT-I, and paramedic-level certifications are issued to students who can meet the registry's examination criteria. There is a national certification available to firefighters. Fire Fighter I or Fire Fighter II are available for fire personnel. In both the EMS and fire examples, practical and written evaluation tools are used. Students must meet a minimum standard of performance, which in these cases, is for a national audience.

State certification examinations are another example of standardized examinations. In EMS, most states teach the EMT-B course by using the U.S. Department of Transportation National Standard Curriculum. Most states use the National Standard Curriculum (NSC) as the basis for their certification examination. The minimum standard of quality is set by the NSC. Many states add supplemental curricula to the examination, but the majority of the examination is formed from the NSC.

In emergency services, other than the semistandardized test, most standardized tests are not for learning purposes. The main purpose is to measure whether a student meets a minimum standard of performance. These examinations have little or no direct feedback on specific questions that are missed. The major learning benefit associated with a standardized examination is the experience of taking the examination.

In contrast, teacher-made examinations are generally reviewed, question by question and the student learns from his mistakes. They are considered a learning tool, in addition to being an evaluation tool.

When looking at the emergency service programs, both forms of examinations have their place in the educational process. Students and instructors should understand the benefits and the drawbacks of the examinations. Instructors must make sure that students know what to expect from each examination format before they take the examination.

Preparing Students for an Examination: A Tale of Two Students

There are two students taking the same examination. Hank has missed classes, not opened the textbook, and has not paid close attention during the class. Floyd works full time, goes to every class session, stays up late at night studying, and worries about the upcoming examination. Hank and Floyd take the examination. Hank finishes the exam first and Floyd finishes next to last. The next week the grades are passed out. Both get basically the same score. Floyd cannot figure out why.

One explanation is that Hank knows how to take the examinations. There is an art to taking examinations, and that art of examination taking should be shared with every student.

Examinations have specific wording patterns. Students who are familiar with these wording patterns can identify the meaning of a question and respond to the question correctly. For example, a student encounters the following multiple-choice question:

During one-rescuer CPR, ventilations for the adult are delivered at the ratio of __?

A. 1 every 5 compressions
B. 2 every 15 compressions
C. 12 per minute
D. 20 per minute

If the student knows how to interpret the question, immediately two answers are eliminated: C and D. Both are not ratios and this leaves only two options, a fifty-fifty chance, at getting the question correct.

The following are test-taking guidelines that should be discussed with all students prior to taking a test:[16]

1. When preparing for an examination, study for short periods of time, days in advance, instead of cramming the night before. Short-term memorization of the information provides only temporary

---

[16]Ibid.

retention of the information. For emergency service personnel, this can mean disaster. Emergency personnel need to know the information all the time, not just for short periods of time.

2. Review all notes, textbook materials, and any study guide materials. Small study groups of three or four people help to discuss the information and encourage retention of the information.

3. Physically prepare for the examination. Attempt to have a stress-free day. Get a good night's sleep the day before the examination. Eat a light meal before the examination. Try to exercise before the examination; increased cardiovascular perfusion provides more blood supply to the brain.

4. Bring examination equipment to the exam. A wristwatch is suggested, so questions can be paced. For example, fifty questions an hour for a multiple-choice test is an average speed. Bring several sharpened pencils. Make sure the lead is dark enough for the examination answer sheets if computer answer sheets are being used. Usually a No. 2 pencil is acceptable. Leave textbooks and notes outside the testing area; they do not provide any benefit at the test.

5. When taking a true/false examination, "absolute answers" like *always, only,* and *never* tend to be *False* statements. "Open answers" like *sometimes* and *maybe* tend to be *True* statements. Look for these key words when reading a question.

6. Multiple-choice questions consist of two parts, a stem and a series of answers. Read the stem and only the stem; some students have found it useful to cover the answer selections with a piece of paper. Find key words and phrases in the stem that identify the answer to the question. Look at the grammar for the question and identify if it is a singular or plural answer format. Then think of the correct answer and look at *all* the answer selections. Only after reading *all* the answers, place the correct answer onto the answer sheet. If your answer does not exactly match the examination answers, begin to eliminate those answers that are totally incorrect. Formulate an educated guess at the answer once the answer possibilities have been reduced by this process of elimination.

7. Use a piece of scrap paper during the examination. Mark down questions that cause concern during the examination. Skip questions that are troublesome and answer them at the end of the examination, time permitting. Remember that studies have shown that your first impression is usually the correct impression. Only change an answer if the first answer is definitely not the right selection.

These guidelines should be shared with students during the first week of a training program, or at least prior to the first significant examination. Having the students perform to the best of their capabilities is what an instructor wants. Knowing how to take an examination can improve a student's performance on the examination.

(Insert the CD-ROM and select the "Test Taking 101" program.)

Test Anxiety

A major contributing factor in a student's performance on an examination may be related to the amount of test anxiety. Test anxiety has psychological and physiological effects. As educational psychologists have found, the amount of test anxiety is directly related to the type of personality traits a student exhibits.

The signs of test anxiety vary among students. Compulsive behaviors or nervousness are commonly observed. Physiological reactions such as frequent urination, sweaty palms, nausea, vomiting, and increased pulse and blood pressure are often observed. The more important the examination, for example, a final or certification examination, the more stressful is the response displayed by the students. Normally anxious students are affected more and actually perform poorly on these types of examinations.[17]

There are ways that an instructor can reduce the amount of test anxiety for students. Specific methods include the following:

1. Adequately prepare the students for taking the examination. State the number of questions for the exam as well as the type of examination format, such as multiple choice, true and false, essay.
2. State the content information being evaluated, for example, specifying Chapters 3, 5, and 6. Knowing what information will be covered helps reduce the fear of the unknown, which is a major contributing factor in test anxiety.
3. Reassure students against the fear of failure. Many students are overwhelmed by this fear. State the percentage of students who pass the examination on the first attempt if this statistic is known. Note if there is a retest option. If this is a modular examination, what is the impact of a poor score on the remaining portion of the course grade?
4. Clearly state the directions for the examination. Remember that when a student is under stress, normal instructions may be misinterpreted. Be specific and repeat important instructions. Students need to be instructed on when to start, how much time is allotted for the examination, and what to do after finishing the examination.
5. Calm the student, in a quiet setting, and explain that this is an opportunity to shine, not a chance for failure.

Instructors must factor an anxiety component into their evaluation of the students. Whether it is a practical or written examination, consider poor performance on an examination due to test anxiety if other objective explanations prove to be unfounded. Test anxiety is a reality and its effects should not be overlooked or underrated.

---

[17]Thomas Good and Jere Brophy. *Educational Psychology: A Realistic Approach* (New York: Holt, Rinehart, and Winston, 1977).

Test Administration

The following are some administration tips when you administer an examination.

PREEXAMINATION ADMINISTRATION

The following administration details need to be addressed before the examination is given:

- Examination starting time.
- Length of time for the exam.
- Examination location. Make sure that the examination area is free of distractions (fire radios, pagers, other classes, hall noise, street noise, etc.). This is especially important for the written examination.
- Room setup. Try to have one chair length between students when possible. Ensure that there is enough space for the examination. Have extra tables and chairs because somehow they always get used.
- Equipment and supplies required for the exam.
- Examination security, for example, numbering exam booklets, writing the examination or scenarios.
- Sufficient copies of the exam.
- Selection or design of answer sheets.
- Scheduling evaluators, victims, and safety personnel for the practical examination.
- Establishing a payment schedule for practical examination personnel.
- Assuring adequate insurance coverage during the examination.
- Formulating the answer key for the examination.
- Designing the evaluation forms for the evaluators.
- Developing a policy for satisfactory and unsatisfactory skill performance.
- Developing the evaluation policies for the examination and the grading of the examination.
- Policies for students caught cheating during the examination.
- Preparing of the students for the examination.

All these administrative details are to be addressed before the examination is given. It is quite a list. Individual instructors add more items, as they see fit, to assure a quality evaluation of the students. Depending upon the type of evaluation tool(s) being used, an instructor may have to perform any or all of these administrative tasks.

ADMINISTRATION DURING THE EXAMINATION

There are numerous administrative tasks that need to be done during the examination. These tasks include the following:

- Greeting the students and assigning seats (open seating, by class, alphabetical).

- Checking in pagers, cellular phones, and radios. Students should be instructed to turn off these devices during the examination due to the distraction that they cause. The potential exists for these devices not only to be a distraction during an exam but also to be a source for coded information.
- Handing out pencils, answer sheets, and scrap paper.
- Taking attendance and assuring admission of students to the examination.
- Completing administrative portions of the answer sheet (name, ID, date, and so on).
- Providing specific instructions for the examination (policy for questions during the exam, time limit for the exam, bathroom excuses, starting the examination, what to do with the completed exam and materials, how to color or write the answers onto the answer sheet, what students should do for ripped or blurred examination copy).
- Setting up an administration area for the return of the examination materials.
- Passing out the examination booklets only when the examination is about to start. For examination security purposes, have each student record the examination booklet number on the answer sheet. When students return the examination materials, count the booklets to assure that all are present and accounted for.
- Monitoring the students during the exam (especially for wandering eyes and cheating). Examination monitors should walk among the students during the exam.
- Observing the students, patient actors, and evaluators during the practical examination.
- Reviewing the practical examination rotation schedule with the students.
- Setting up the makeup area.
- Having evaluator sign in. Assure that all evaluation personnel sign time sheets for reimbursement.

Individual instructors develop and use these and other administrative policies in their examinations. Every instructor needs to use policies that will ensure a quality examination.

Alternative Forms of Evaluation

In addition to the traditional forms of evaluation, technological advancements have made it possible to enhance the assessment of a student's knowledge. Technological advancements have greatly improved the ways students are assessed. Advancements include the following:

1. Videotaping of skill sessions
2. Computer-generated test questions
3. Computer-video interactive programming
4. Computer-based examinations

VIDEOTAPING OF SKILL SESSIONS

Professional athletes videotape their performances so that they can review their mistakes and improve their performance. This same approach can be used for skill instruction in any emergency service program.

The availability of VCR cameras places this form of technology within the reach of most instructors and training institutes. Instructors can videotape the performance of students at a skill station. Following completion of the skill, the students and the instructor watch the videotaped presentation. Positive and negative aspects are reviewed and are discussed. This technique is useful for students who are having difficulties learning a specific skill. Often, visually seeing themselves making the mistakes is enough of a learning experience to correct the procedures the next time the skill is performed.

The equipment needed for videotaping a skill session includes

- Video camera and tripod
- TV/VCR
- Sufficient blank videotapes

Position the camera where it will show most of the active skill assessments. Using a tripod reduces unnecessary camera motion. If the skill, such as a rope traverse across a river, requires different camera angles, handheld videotaping should be used. While taping, vary the shots from wide to close, especially when specific skills are being performed.

The video camera is a powerful skill development training adjunct. Its use must be prefaced with close instructor observation and guidance. Videotaping of skill sessions is *not* intended for disciplinary reasons; for example, "You screwed up and I am going to show you where." When used for its intended purpose, it can be a tremendous adjunct to a training program.

COMPUTER-GENERATED TEST QUESTIONS

This evaluation adjunct can lessen the amount of preparation time for an instructor. Many textbooks now come with a computer-generated examination. Through the use of this computer program, an instructor can choose questions from different formats and construct a written examination. Not only is the examination written, but most programs provide an answer sheet and an answer key.

There are numerous independent computer test banks from which an instructor can create an examination. Having these computer test banks greatly reduces the amount of preparation time for an examination. The instructor needs only to review the questions in the bank and select those that will fit into their examination format.

Another feature offered by some computer test banks is the ability for instructors to design their own examination questions and include them in the test bank. Specific objectives and page references are usually required for a test bank. The instructor's questions can be referenced right along with the computer test bank questions. This gives an examination the best of both worlds, semistandardized examination questions as well as instructor-made questions.

There are pitfalls associated with computer test banks. Many of the test bank questions have never been regionally or nationally studied for their reliability and validity. Thus, close review is suggested when selecting questions from test banks. Make sure there is only *one* correct answer and that the answer coincides with the lesson material. Test banks that do not have specific references to the lesson objectives should be avoided.

A working knowledge of computers is useful, but is not necessary for most test banks. Simply follow the display screen instructions and use the help screens that are provided in most programs. Select the questions that you want and then print them. Review the examination for any mistakes. If everything is all right, copy enough examination books and answer sheets for the class.

Computer test banks can be a valuable tool. Not all questions and answers may be correct for your class. The time saving in designing an examination can be tremendous for an instructor. Test banks have become a major asset in the preparation of examination materials for many instructors. Through the use of these test banks and the instructor's own questions, students are given "the best of both worlds."

COMPUTER-VIDEO INTERACTIVE PROGRAMMING

Long used by industry for training and retraining of personnel, this form of educational programming is rapidly growing throughout emergency service training programs. A major use of this program format is for evaluation purposes.

As opposed to a student reading a scenario from a piece of paper and responding to a series of questions, the use of a computer interactive learning system creates a real-life scenario that is displayed onto a computer video screen. The computer displays options for the resolution of the scenario. At each step, the program only proceeds after the student selects an option. The video session ends with a resolution to the scenario, whether it has a positive or negative outcome.

The system requires minimal to no computer training on the part of the student. Touch monitor screens and a mouse make the interface with the computer system minimal on the student's part. The computer–video interactive system consists of a PC computer, color monitor, laser-disc player, and the laser-disc/software. Simple screen command instructions make it possible for a student to have a one-on-one training session with the computer.

Skill-sensored CPR and intubation manikins are connected to the PC computer and laser disc. At specific segments of the program, the student is asked to perform CPR, ventilation, or to intubate. The student's performance is rated against the AHA standards. Based upon the student's performance, actual certification can be issued by the monitoring instructor.

The computer–video interactive programming is only one aspect of the interactive learning process. The interactive programming provides an alternative to traditional types of evaluations. Through the use of real situations created by the computer, a student's decision skills can be assessed. Chapter 12 has additional information on computer–video interactive programming and other forms of interactive programming.

COMPUTER-BASED EXAMINATIONS

With the advances in computer software, computer-based examinations can be easily created and administered. Instead of using the paper or pen test, students take their examination on the computer.

Advantages to these examinations include:

- Selection of various examination formats
- Inclusion of color images, graphics, and animations (assessment of a heart rate or blood pressure)
- Easily and instantly corrected by the computer
- Immediate feedback to the student regarding their performance; can tell students why a question was not correct
- Allows for variable time of completion; with Internet access, can be taken online
- Depending on the software, relatively easy to create and modify questions
- Improves classroom time and allows more time to be focused on the lesson material and less time on the examinations

Disadvantages include:

- Instructor's learning curve and familiarity with computers and interactive examination software
- Student's access, familiarity, and acceptance of computers and these types of exams
- Initial costs of computers, software, training of faculty, and similar items
- Software limits on the types of question formats that can be used
- Immediate feedback can intimidate some students. After missing several questions in a row, students can get the feeling that they are failing the examination. Software needs to allow immediate or delayed feedback.

An impressive aspect of the computer-based examination is the immediacy of the feedback to the students. The feedback can be written to identify why an answer was not correct. This allows students to learn while they are taking the examination. A database keeps track of the correct and incorrect responses. At the end of the exam, the student can print out the results. The instructor, through a variety of methods, can access the same database. These include direct download, e-mail, or via the Internet.

(Insert the CD-ROM and click on the file marked Gameinst.)

Summary

By now, it is clear that an instructor has an unlimited source of evaluation tools that can be used to assess a student's learning development. The key is for the instructor to know when to use each of the tools.

The role of the behavioral objectives and Bloom's *Taxonomy of Educational Objectives* were related several times over. They are the foundation for any form of evaluation. The difficulty of the examination can be directly determined by both factors. When creating an examination, these two indicators must be looked at first before any questions are written.

Oral questions, practical evaluations, and written examinations were identified in this chapter. Through the use of real examination examples, each form of evaluation tool was dissected into specific components. Each tool has a specific purpose. Instructors need to select the right tool for the job, in this case, the right tool for the lesson objectives. Psychomotor objectives cannot be evaluated through oral or written questions. Choosing the right tool is essential.

The administration of an evaluation is not a simple process. Many components must be prepared before an evaluation. Policies for the exam, check sheets, examination copies, and so on are all components that must be established before the evaluation can begin. Then during the evaluation, additional administrative procedures are needed to assure a valid examination.

Test anxiety is often overlooked during examinations. Test anxiety has real physiological and psychological effects upon students. Realization of these effects is a key observation that must be made by the instructor. This factor needs to be taken into account when reviewing the performance of a group of students.

Evaluation is a necessary component in the education process. Learning is invisible, but changes in a student's behavior are not invisible. Without evaluation tools, an instructor would have no means to tell if a student has learned the material. No single evaluation tool tells the whole learning potential of a student. Only after multiple forms of evaluation tools are used does an instructor really know if a student has learned the information.

Chapter 11

Program Evaluation

➤ **OBJECTIVES**

- Define *quality improvement* as it pertains to education.
- Identify the importance of accountability in education.
- Identify the basic components of an examination analysis to include the following:
  —Item analysis
  —Item difficulty
  —Basic examination statistics
  —Developing grades for the students
- Develop course evaluation forms that address the following categories:
  —Student opinions
  —Instructor performance
  —Course coordination/administration
  —Institute/facilities
- Formulate a strategy to evaluate the whole program, as well as the specific components.
- Translate the results of the evaluation into actions.
- Identify the need to keep an open mind when performing a program evaluation.

Chapter 10 presented the tools that an instructor uses to assess a student's change in behavior, that is, learning. No one single tool gave the whole learning perspective. The same holds true for a program evaluation. No one evaluation tool provides the entire picture of a training program's overall performance.

This chapter deals with a subject that is often overlooked, misunderstood, and incorrectly interpreted. There are tools used in a program evaluation that are quality improvement oriented. There are other tools that are statistically oriented, opinion oriented, and objective oriented. All assess the performance of the course, which is the primary purpose of conducting a program evaluation.

A program evaluation is designed not only to identify strengths and weaknesses in a course but also to assess student attitudes. These both lead to program enhancements.

The approaches used to assess a program's effectiveness vary from institute to institute. Some institutes use the final examination results as the benchmark for the assessment of a program's effectiveness. Others use student opinion survey forms to assess the program. In many institutes, a course coordinator monitors the actual instruction and rates the instructor's performance. And, unfortunately, many institutes have no form of program evaluation.

This chapter will identify the basic concepts associated with a program evaluation. Specific details from each of these areas will be discussed. No one assessment tool gives a "total picture." Using those tools that are appropriate for emergency service programs are the perspectives discussed in this chapter.

Accountability

In life, everyone is responsible for something (Figure 11-1). Whether it is to their job, family, children, church, or community, everyone shares a degree of responsibility. Education is no different. When students attain a good education, it is the result of everyone's work (instructors, course coordinators, and program administrators). Conversely, when students attain a poor learning experience, everyone's work in the institute is assessed to identify the problem(s) that caused the poor experience. Developing a program evaluation to observe the results of the learning experience is being accountable. Being accountable is important, but it is not the whole reason for conducting a program evaluation. Another factor is the quality of the educational experience.

Quality

According to *Webster's New World Dictionary*, the term *quality* has this educational meaning: *"the degree of excellence which a thing possesses."*[1] Quality improvement (QI) plays a key role in program evaluation. In part, the reason for performing a program evaluation is to assess the degree of excellence that has been achieved during a program. Student performance and the overall program performance are reviewed in a comprehensive quality improvement program.

The main emphasis of a QI program is to determine the degree of excellence and to assess how to improve the process. To help determine this perspective, two viewpoints are assessed: an internal and an external viewpoint. The internal viewpoint is designed to look at the institute's objectives: "How did the program measure up?" and "Were the goals met?" These types of probing questions are asked during an internal review. The external viewpoint is gained from the students, or from the community that is served by the program. Students' opinions and impressions about a program are reviewed: "Did the program meet your expectations?" and "What did you like or dislike about the program?" Questions such as these provide the institute with information about the program from an outside viewpoint.

The following chart outlines factors that are assessed during a program:

---

[1]*From Webster's New World™ College Dictionary, 4th Edition.* Copyright © 2000, 1999 by Hungry Minds, Inc. All rights reserved. Reproduced here by permission of the publisher.

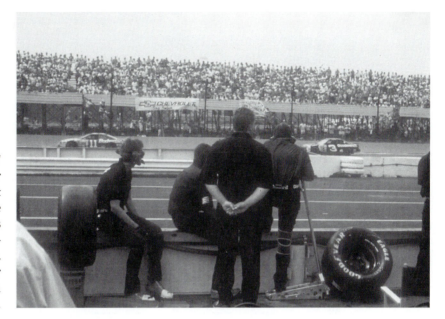

Figure 11-1
The racing car driver depends upon the pit crew to service the car in as little time as possible. To accomplish this objective, each crew member is responsible for a particular job.

- Performance
- Reliability or consistency
- Facilities/equipment
- Reputation of the program
- Conformance with standards
- Response to needs of the students/community at large

These six factors help to measure the status of the program. These factors determine the quality improvement evaluation.

The quality improvement evaluation is a continual process. Figure 11-2 illustrates the process that is used in a quality improvement program. A key aspect of a program assessment is to evaluate throughout the whole course, not just at the end of the course. As is suggested by the diagram, the designation of certain areas of assessment should be included in the program assessment. Any of the six quality factors can be assessed during the program. Assessments during the program allow any potential errors to be identified and corrected before the course ends.

This chapter provides a detailed approach for designing a quality improvement program. Each section provides specific components that are used in the overall assessment.

The Objectives

We are back at the construction site. A construction worker cannot effectively construct a building unless there is a set of detailed blueprints to follow. As shown with a lesson plan, the behavioral objectives are the blueprints for the entire lesson. The same concept holds true with the assessment of a training program. Specific goals and directions are established, before the assessment of a program occurs.

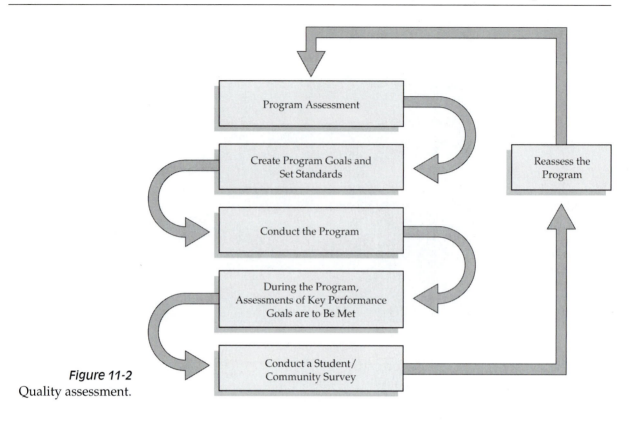

Figure 11-2
Quality assessment.

The objectives for the program evaluation differ from those used to write lesson plans. An individual lesson plan plots the degree of behavioral change for the students. A program evaluation looks at the level of proficiency that the students, instructors, and administrators have attained. Specific program goals are set for each category. These goals are not only assessed when the program ends, but are assessed during the program. Assessments made during the program help to gauge where the institute stands in respect to its program goals.

The goals that are established must meet two key criteria:

1. The goals must be measurable.
2. The goals must be attainable—those that can be reached.

The following are examples of program objectives:

A. Upon completion of the EMT basic training program, the course final written examination will be administered. Minimum passing score for the examination is 75%, with an ideal class average of 80%.
B. All classroom areas will be free from outside distractions.
C. Instructors will provide a 10-minute break every 1 to 1 ½ hours of classroom instruction.
D. The course coordinator will be present for at least 85% of the class sessions.

Often, goals are set too high for the type of courses/students being taught. Yet there are other program goals that cannot be evaluated. The examples just outlined are all capable of being evaluated. For example, item A can be assessed by statistical review of the examination results, items B and C are assessed by a student survey, and item D is assessed by an administrative review of time sheets.

Program goals are to be written before the program starts. Ideally, several months before a program starts, a group of instructors and course administrators needs to develop the institute's goals for a particular time period, for example, specific courses, half year, and full year. Many training institutes develop long-range program goals. Having a clear direction of where a program is supposed to be headed, helps everyone in the institute better understand where their own performance, and those of their students, are headed.

The Strategy

The reason for the program evaluation is to evaluate the whole program. There are numerous components to an educational program. The strategy, or the plan of action, is the first item to identify. The strategy is developed at the same time the program's objectives are being written. The objectives identify the educational components that are being assessed. The strategy identifies how the objectives are assessed. It is the strategy that identifies the evaluation tools that are used to attain the information.

As seen in the assessment of student performance, there are evaluation tools used to assess both knowledge and skills. In a program evaluation, the evaluation tools measure specific types of information. There are statistical evaluation tools used to assess examination performance. Student survey forms are used to assess opinions. Another type of survey is a forecasting survey, which is sent to the community at large. This type of survey is useful for identifying future training needs, and assessing the reputation of the institute. Each tool provides different types of information. Only after reviewing all the information can any conclusions be reached regarding the final evaluation.

EXAMINATION ANALYSIS

One of the most common areas that educators look at when assessing an institute's or program's quality is the written examination scores. The written examination is designed to objectively assess the degree of learning that has occurred. Since the examination is based upon the course curriculum or textbook, it is one of the first indicators that is reviewed.

Often the examination is not the best indicator, nor should it be the first indicator to be reviewed. If an institute is designing a total quality improvement program, the assessment should be based on other indicators besides the written examination performance. These can include monitored performance evaluations of the instructors, opinion surveys of the students, or the review of course coordinator reports regarding student grievances.

The specific examination tools that will be addressed in this section include:

1. Item analysis of the examination
2. Identification of the item difficulty for the examination
3. Identification of the distribution of student scores
4. Validation of the examination results
5. Assessment of the examination's reliability
6. Development of grade formats for the students

These tools assess how effective the student's learning experience and written examination performance were in objective terms.

Item Analysis

Not all examinations measure what they are supposed to. Questions are often misworded or miskeyed or simply do not contain the correct answer. A bad examination can lead to incorrect information regarding the student's learning. There are often questions that are not incorrect, but after looking at how the students responded to a question, an alternate answer may be apparent. Performing an item analysis of the examination can assess all these types of situations.[2]

An item analysis is a listing of each student's answer to a particular question. The example looks at an analysis from a class of twenty students. The examination is from a multiple-choice examination. In Table 11-1, several answers cause concern. Less than 50 percent of the students answered items 2, 3, and 5 correctly. Each of these questions should be individually reviewed for any miskeyed answers, sentence structure problems, grammar, misspelling, or no real answer to the question. There is some reason for students missing more than 50 percent of the items. Item 4 raises a different concern: Is the question too easy? It too should be reviewed. Has the answer been given away by another question in the examination? Or does the question give away the answer because of a grammatical error? These are the kinds of questions that are asked when a high percentage of students gets a particular question correct.

What should an instructor do when an item is found to be incorrect by the item analysis? All the scores for the examination should be adjusted to reflect a question's inaccuracy. One method is to drop the question from the examination and recalculate the scores based on a new total score. The question should be withdrawn and modified before it is used again.

An item analysis should be done on every examination. Each class is different. The analysis can indicate if the students understood the course material. The wealth of information provided by the item analysis makes it worth the time it takes to create the analysis.

---

[2]Gilbert Sax. *Principles of Education and Psychological Measurement and Evaluation*, 3rd ed. (Belmont, Calif.: Wadsworth, 1989).

Table 11-1. Sample Test Item Analysis

Item No.	A	B	C	D	E
1.	0	2	10*	3	5
2.	2	2	8	8*	0
3.	1	5*	4	6	4
4.	0	0	2	17*	1
5.	4	8*	4	3	1

* = Correct answer

Item Difficulty

Linked to the item analysis is a process for determining a question's difficulty. In Chapter 10, one way of determining the question's difficulty was to use the *Taxonomy of Educational Objectives*. Using the taxonomy provides a baseline for the anticipated performance on a question. During the examination analysis, an exact item difficulty score can be identified.

It is measured by using the item analysis. In Table 11-2, titled "Sample Test Item Analysis with Item Difficulty," another column has been added to the previous item analysis. Looking at the number of correct answers (*CA*) for each item in the analysis, and then dividing it by the total number of students (*N*) equals the item difficulty (*ID*).[3]

$$CA/N = ID$$

A high item-difficulty score means that it is an easy question. Conversely, a low item-difficulty score is a difficult question. Identification of the item difficulty can improve an examination for future use. This is possible because the item difficulty can be linked to the test blueprint. For each question, an item difficulty score can be identified. When it comes time to modify an examination, the instructor can look at the item difficulty score and insert a new question with a similar item difficulty score. This allows the examination blueprint to remain nearly unchanged.

The ideal examination is one in which there are balanced item difficulty scores. As a general guideline, any item that has an item difficulty score *below .55* should be reviewed for question validity. At .55, almost half the group answered the item incorrectly. An examination that has questions with an item difficulty score of *.60 through .95* and has a normal distribution of scores is considered to be a balanced examination.

Balancing the question difficulty using an item difficulty analysis is a clear-cut way of determining the actual item performance for each question. As an examination is used repeatedly, a sense of how a class should perform on the examination can be predicted. This enables the instructor to look at the performance of one class versus another class. The comparison

---

[3]Ibid.

Item No.	A	B	C	D	E	ID
1.	0	2	10*	3	5	.50
2.	2	2	8	8*	0	.40
3.	1	5*	4	6	4	.25
4.	0	0	2	17*	1	.85
5.	4	8*	4	3	1	.40

Table 11-2. Sample Test Item Analysis with Item Difficulty (N = 20)

* = Correct answer

between the two classes allows the instructor to gauge each class's performance for a particular point in its training. Changes can be based from this comparison if deficiencies are noted between the two classes.

Item difficulty is a powerful tool to evaluate each question on an examination. Instructors should realize its usefulness and routinely analyze examination questions. The objective information provided is invaluable in determining the validity of the examination.

Statistics for Examinations

Looking at a listing of the students' scores easily identifies how a class performed on an examination. There is a wealth of statistical information that can be attained by looking at a group of students' scores. Some of the basic statistics that an instructor should review include:

1. Distribution of the scores
2. Average scores
3. Examination reliability

These statistics are very basic and are considered a starting point, when looking at an examination's overall performance. Let's look at each one of these areas separately.

DISTRIBUTION OF SCORES

There are many ways of viewing information. Take, for example, any news event. You could read about it in the morning newspaper, hear about it on the radio, or see and hear the event on television. Viewing examination scores is similar to viewing a news event. There are countless ways to show the scores. The following examples are considered to be the basic principles for reporting examination results.

The first distribution is a listing of high to low scores in one column. Then, beside each score, create a second column that lists the number of students that attained the score on the examination. An example of this distribution is shown in Table 11-3. This distribution appears to have scores clustered around 5–7. This list of numbers is not easily visualized. If the

Table 11-3.	Test A. Ten-Point Quiz, 15 Students
Scores	*No. Students*
10	1
9	0
8	2
7	4
6	3
5	2
4	1
3	0
2	2
1	0
0	0

numbers are placed onto a chart, this will provide a visual description of the students scores. Recording the scores on a chart is a common method for showing how well students performed (Figure 11-3).

Educators like to see a perfect distribution of scores from an examination. The perfect distribution of scores is referred to as the normal distribution. A normal distribution has the majority of the scores centered around the average score for the examination. The mean, or average score, should be positioned in the center of the distribution. In ideal circumstances, 95 percent of the class should have scores within the major area covered by the distribution. This leaves only 2.5 percent on each side of the curve for extremely high and low scores. Figure 11-4 shows the normal curve.

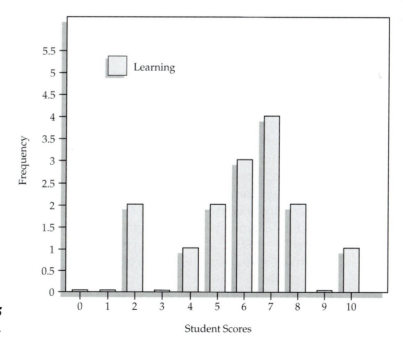

Figure 11-3
Test A.

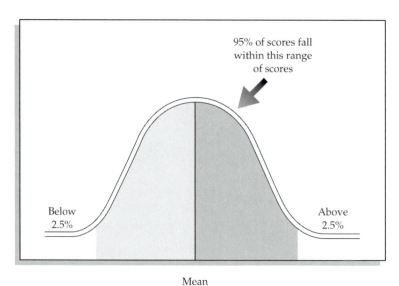

Figure 11-4
Normal distribution
table.

In practical applications, the normal distribution is not the rule but the exception. Most examination distributions do not conform to the normal distribution. They can be off in one direction: Either the distribution is to the high side or to the low side. Often, there can be such a variety of scores that there is no clustering of the scores. Whenever these situations occur, the distribution is said to be skewed. There are two specific skews that are important to an instructor: Positive skew and negative skew.[4] See Figure 11-5 for examples.

The information from these skewed distributions can immediately alert an instructor to a potential problem with an examination. The positive skew example shows very few scores toward the top of the distribution, and the majority of the scores are below the mean. Interpreting the chart reveals potential causes for the distribution. One cause may have been that the examination was too difficult for the majority of the class. To determine this, look at the individual student scores. Look, especially, at the students who were performing exceedingly well before the exam and those who were performing poorly before the test. Compare their performance on the examination. If the individuals who were expected to do well on the examination actually did poorly, this could be an indicator that the examination may have been too difficult.

A negative skew has the opposite effect from a positive skew. In a negative distribution, the majority of the students are above the mean. An immediate interpretation is that the examination was too easy. Only a few individuals scored poorly on the examination. A negative distribution needs to have the same investigative review as seen with the positive skew. An instructor needs to review the scores and to validate the examination results. If an examination has overevaluated or underevaluated a student's knowledge, this examination has not represented the amount of learning for a group of students. For this reason, instructors should routinely review the distribution results.

---

[4]Ibid.

Positive Skewed Distribution

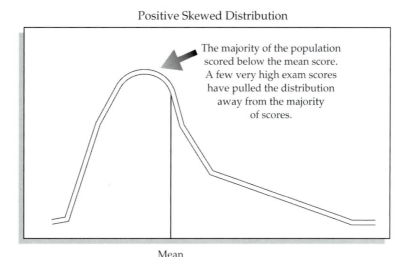

The majority of the population scored below the mean score. A few very high exam scores have pulled the distribution away from the majority of scores.

Mean

Negative Skewed Distribution

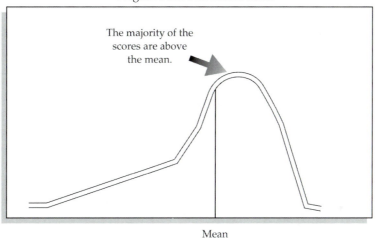

The majority of the scores are above the mean.

Figure 11-5
Positive and negative distribution curves.

Mean

AVERAGE SCORES

One of the average scores was already mentioned, the mean, or average score. When someone mentions average score, the mean is the first score that comes to mind. To a statistician, an average score has several different definitions. The same statistician will also state that the mean score, by itself, is considered to be a raw piece of data that needs to be viewed cautiously.

This section looks at three methods for measuring the average score of an examination. These three methods are considered "raw" measurements. There are other statistical measures that can be used to identify the exact position of each student's score. The average scores that are discussed are:

1. Mean
2. Mode
3. Median

For an instructor to assess the true average score for an examination, all three measurements need to be assessed. In a normal distribution, all three should be the center line that divides the distribution. In a skewed distribution, each may have a different line location within the distribution. An instructor should use the measurement that best represents the distribution of the student's score.

Mean

The most commonly used measurement for the average score is the mean. It is attained by adding up all the scores from the examination and dividing by the total number of students that took the examination:

$$\text{Total scores}/\text{Number of students} = \text{Mean}$$

This is a crude estimate of how the students performed on the examination. As seen with skewed distributions, the mean does not reflect all the students' scores. One or two extremely high or low scores will raise or lower the mean. The mean will move with the extreme scores and will not reflect the majority of the students. For this reason, an instructor should not use the mean as the only measurement. The mode and median also need to be assessed.[5]

Mode

The mode is defined as the most commonly occurring score in the examination. To determine the mode, count the number of student scores for each examination score. *The largest number of single examination scores is the mode.* If the majority of student scores are clustered in a distribution, the likelihood of the mode appearing in the cluster is high. If the distribution is skewed, it may appear anywhere. In a very large distribution, there may be multiple modes.[6] Figure 11-6 shows the mean and the mode for a distribution of exam scores.

Referencing Table 11-4, the mean is the more reflective average score for the distribution. Over 11 students attained at least the mean, where only 4 students were at a score of 18. The mode does not reflect all the student scores for this distribution.

Median Score

The median score is a more involved measurement than the previous two. The median score is the exact score in the middle of the distribution. It is based upon a percentage from the total number of students taking the examination. To calculate the median score, the first step is to create a column called a "cumulative frequency" (cf). The cumulative frequency is formed by adding up the number of student scores at each level. The top value is to equal the actual number of students who took the examination. Then, each cumulative score is divided by the total number of students taking the

---

[5]From *Statistics for the Behavioral Sciences A First Course for, 3rd edition*, by F. Gravetter and L Wallnau © 1998. Reprinted with permission of Wadsworth, an imprint of the Wadsworth Group, a division of Thomson Learning. Fax 800 730-2215.
[6]Ibid.

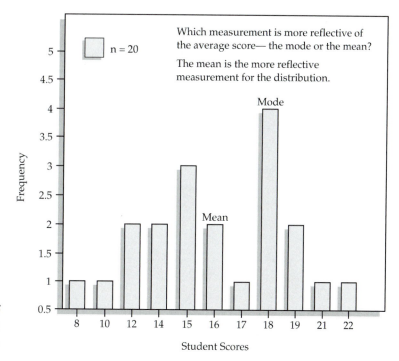

Which measurement is more reflective of the average score— the mode or the mean?

The mean is the more reflective measurement for the distribution.

Figure 11-6
Examination results
for 20 students.

examination. The score that is at the 50 percent indicator is called the median score.

Let's add the median score to the previous example (Table 11-5).[7] The c% column, to many educators, is referred to as a percentile. Percentiles show student scores based on a 100 percent scale. Notice that the median score is between the scores of 15 and 16. There is a statistical method for determining the exact score. For the purpose of this example, it is important to note that the mean and the median are nearly identical. Thus, for the

Table 11-4.   25-Point Exam, 20 Students

Scores	Score Frequency
22	1
21	1
19	2
18	4 (Mode)
17	1
16	2 (Mean)
15	3
14	2
12	2
10	1
8	1

---
[7]Ibid.

Scores	Score Frequency	cf	c%
			Table 11-5. Median Score
22	1	20	100%
21	1	19	95%
19	2	18	90%
18	4 (Mode)	16	80%
17	1	12	60%
16	2 (Mean)	11	55% Median (15–16)
15	3	9	45%
14	2	6	30%
12	2	4	20%
10	1	2	10%
8	1	1	5%

distribution, using either the mean or the median score would be equally reflective of the actual average score for the distribution.[8]

Identifying the true average scores assists the instructor in locating the correct average for the distribution. As was noted, the mean can be affected by one or two high or low scores. To find the true average score requires all three measures to be assessed and compared. Then, the instructor can select the measurement that best reflects the average score for the distribution.

EXAMINATION RELIABILITY

Statisticians use various measurements for determining if an examination is reliable. They make these measurements to evaluate if the examination has consistency among the questions. Through the use of a mathematical formula, a determination of the examination's reliability is made.

One of the more frequently used formulas is the Kuder–Richardson reliability formula (Exhibit 11-1). It determines the internal consistency of the examination. The scoring range is from 0 to 1. An examination is said to be reliable at .60 and higher.[9]

Educators also measure an examination's reliability by repeated administrations of an examination. Theoretically, if an examination is given to a group of students one week, and the same examination is given to the same students a week later, the scores should be nearly identical. Emergency service instructors would not perform this type of educational test in their classes. However, an instructor should keep track of an examination's performance each time it is administered. Although different students are taking the examination, if the material presented in the course is the same,

---

[8]Ibid.

[9]G. Frederick Kuder and M. W. Richardson. *The Theory of the Estimation of Test Reality*, University of North Carolina at Greensboro, Greensboro, N.C. : Psychometrika Vol. 2 (September 1937).

Exhibit 11-1

Kuder-Richardson Formula #21

$$Kr21 = \left(\frac{n}{n-1}\right) \quad 1 - \left(\frac{M - \frac{(M)}{n}}{SD}\right)$$

To complete the formula you need only to know the following:

n = no. exam items

M = Mean

SD squared

$n = 50 \quad M = 38 \quad SD$ squared $= 35$

$$Kr21 = \frac{50}{49} \qquad\qquad 1 - \left(\frac{38 - \frac{(38)\,sq}{50}}{35}\right)$$

$$= 1.02 \qquad\qquad 1 - \left(\frac{38 - \frac{1444}{50}}{35}\right)$$

$$= 1.02 \qquad\qquad 1 - \left(\frac{38 - 28.88}{35}\right)$$

$$= 1.02 \qquad\qquad 1 - \left(\frac{9.12}{35}\right)$$

$$= 1.02 \qquad\qquad (1 - .260) = (.74)$$

the scores on the examination should be similar. This can be a factor to look at when evaluating a program.

Instructors should check the reliability of their examinations. Assessing the examination reliability is part of assuring a valid measurement of a student's learning experience.

GRADES FOR THE STUDENTS

Typical adult learners enroll in emergency service training programs to attain information. These adult learners are not necessarily motivated by grades, but are motivated by the desire to learn new information, so they can better perform their daily jobs.[10] Still, there are other adult learners who are concerned with obtaining good grades. Thus, for all adult learners, an instructor needs to provide a fair grading system.

Once the instructor completes the item analysis and statistical review, the individual student scores can be calculated. When an instructor assigns

---

[10]Malcolm Knowles. *The Adult Learner: A Neglected Species* (Houston, Tex.: Gulf, 1990).

a score, the instructor can use one or two scoring categories, either a letter grade or a numerical score. The letter score (A, B, C, D, F) is probably more familiar to most adult learners. The numerical score (4, 3, 2, 1 or 95, 90, 85, 80, . . .) is closely associated with higher learning institutes, for example, post-high-school or college. The instructor needs to clearly identify one of the categories in the beginning of the class. In either category, the passing score for the course or examination is to be identified during the first class session.

Grades for practical examinations have already been identified in Chapter 10. Most adult learners do not easily accept the term *failure*. A term like *unsatisfactory* is better. Unsatisfactory is interpreted as not meeting the accepted criteria at that specific time; failure carries with it the notion that no aspect of a student's performance was correct. Chances are only a single segment or element was performed incorrectly. But a student usually does not know that. Unsatisfactory and satisfactory scoring scales should be the preferred terms for adult learners.

Whether it is a practical or written examination, the instructor must maintain a consistent scoring system. Some students will use scores as a competitive gauge to better their own personal performance. Overall, the majority of students will use the scores as a gauge to see their individual position in the class. Their main motivation is not grade performance but information retention. Gaining information to better themselves and to better perform their jobs is their motivation force. Grades are secondary to knowledge. Instructors should recognize this characteristic of adult learners.[11]

Developing the Course Evaluation

One method for assessing whether a program has achieved its established goals is to ask the students and faculty objective questions. Responses to these questions help to identify how the institute is meeting the goals. Another approach is to observe the students, instructors, and administration. This approach has a degree of subjectivity that impacts the final results. However, when combined with a survey and a review of the program's statistics, the subjectivity is reduced.

This section looks at both the development of a survey and at the construction of performance-based observations. Both are valuable evaluation tools to use in a program evaluation.

SURVEYS

Four elements should be evaluated in the survey approach:

1. Student opinions
2. Instructor viewpoints
3. Course coordinator/administration views
4. The institute/facilities

---

[11]Ibid.

The survey could be a comprehensive form that asks questions from each of the four categories. Or the survey can be specifically geared to each category. This second approach is more time consuming, but it provides better information.

The survey is an aspect of the program evaluation strategy. With the development of the evaluation strategy comes the development of specific surveys that will be used. Since this is an overall program evaluation, the questions are directly associated with an established goal or standard for the institute.

Rating Scales

Several rating scales may be used in surveys. The most commonly used scales are the numerical rating scale and the graphic rating scale. The numerical scale is the simplest type. The following is an example:

5 = Outstanding
4 = Above average
3 = Average
2 = Fair
1 = Poor

1. The primary instructor's preparation of course material was . . .
   1   2   3   4   5
2. The quality of the audiovisual materials was . . .
   1   2   3   4   5

A program administrator can quickly tally the information and identify the common trends and opinions expressed in the survey. If, for example, there were two surveys, one designed for students and the other designed for instructors, it would be appropriate to assess the same objectives for both surveys. A comparison of the responses to the same objective from two different perspectives can be assessed. The numerical rating scale would make this type of comparison very easy to identify since specific values are listed on the rating scale.

The graphic rating scale is not as defined as the numeric. It uses a line graph to plot the opinions to a specific question. Exhibit 11-2 is an example of a graphic rating scale: With this rating scale, it is possible to obtain values between a given value (e.g., 3.3, 4.5, 2.3). Instead of locking a respondent into a

Exhibit 11-2

Graphic Rating Scale				
Too Much		Adequate		Too Little
5	4	3	2	1

1. How much practice time was allotted during class?

specific number, a specific value assessment for a question can be attained. For tally purposes, this rating scale is much more difficult to calculate. However, the information is more a true reflection of the actual opinions for the question.

A variation of the two rating scales is the multiple-choice rating scale. Written on the same format as a multiple-choice examination, specific answers are preidentified. The respondent selects the answer that meets his or her opinions. On a typical form, four answers are preidentified and a fifth answer left blank. When the respondents feel that the preidentified answers do not reflect their opinion, they can write in the response. The following is an example of a multiple-choice survey:

1. The audiovisual materials that were used during the program were

    _____.

    a. Poor. Most were old and outdated. They did not enhance the course material.
    b. Fair. A few of the AV materials were outdated, but overall they complemented the lesson material.
    c. Good. The materials were current and enhanced the lesson materials.
    d. Excellent. Greatly enhanced the course materials.
    e. (Write in the response on the attached form.)

The multiple-choice survey is very easy to tally. The questions can be reworded to allow a comparison between two different categories, for example, students and instructors. The preselected responses allow a respondent who is not familiar with educational concepts to respond to the question. The downside to preselected responses is that the survey author is pointing a respondent toward a conclusion that may not totally reflect the individual's opinion. The respondent often selects the answer only because he does not want to write in a response. Care must be used when observing the results of a multiple-choice survey.

Survey Questions

The key to a successful survey is the way the questions are written on the survey form and interpreted by the person completing the survey. Program evaluation questions are based upon accepted educational concepts or upon an accepted curriculum. In other words, the goals for a program become the evaluation mechanism for the program.

Each question covers a specific goal. The question is to be written in simple English. Just like written examination questions, a program evaluation question should be a complete sentence whenever possible. Remembering these concepts can increase the validity of the survey.

Survey Format

The following basic guidelines are used by most surveys.

1. The overall survey should appear simple, not overwhelming. Many surveys are too complex in their appearance. The respondent should be able to look at the survey and easily identify the information being requested.

2. The questions must be written to the point. There is no need for fancy terms or lengthy sentences. The questions for a survey are based upon accepted educational objectives or accepted standards. Refer back to the previous section dealing with survey questions.

3. There should be only one rating scale. This will lessen the respondent's confusion as to which rating scale is being used for a particular section.

4. Write the rating scale at the top section of each page of the survey. If the rating scale has the scale built into each question, for example, in graphic type, then the respondents have all the information they need right in front of them.

5. The respondent should remain anonymous. As seen in Chapter 10 for essay examinations, one of the key factors for increasing the validity of the examination is to hide the name of the student. This helps protect the examination from subjectivity. The same subjectivity can influence a survey. Thus a survey should not request the name of the respondent.[12]

6. A sound survey is a reflection of the survey's directions. Students or faculty members often complete surveys with no monitor present to clarify a particular question. The directions to a survey must contain enough details so that anyone who completes the survey can do so without difficulty. Poor directions result in poor information, as the respondent, if unsure or confused, will provide inaccurate information. This invalidates some of the information for the survey.

The use of these guidelines not only helps in writing a survey, but can lead to improved validity for the survey. A survey is constructed to assess the opinions from a group of individuals. From this survey, key programming decisions will be made. If a survey has inaccurately assessed the individuals, then the decisions being made will be in error. Care must be used when developing, using, and evaluating with a survey. The information attained from a survey should be helpful, not harmful.

The survey can only provide opinions from the respondents. Often, this information is not enough to base program changes on. Another evaluation tool, a performance evaluation, can provide more substantial information. The next section looks at the design and use of performance evaluations.

PERFORMANCE EVALUATIONS

A performance evaluation is a tool that can provide more in-depth information than is possible to attain on a survey alone. The categories are the same as those for the surveys. Performance evaluations can be conducted for each of the following groups:

1. Students
2. Instructors

---

[12]William J. Mehrens and Irvin J. Lehmann. *Measurement and Evaluation in Education and Psychology* (New York: Holt, Rinehart and Winston, 1978).

3. Course administration
4. Facilities

The difference between a performance evaluation and a survey is that a trained evaluator physically monitors each group. The monitor uses preprepared objective-based check sheets. As with the survey approach, these objectives are based upon the broad goals for the institute.

The approach used to evaluate students' performing skills is the same as that used in the program evaluation. The same pitfalls are also carried over (e.g., the halo effect, subjectivity, and poor evaluators). As with any educational evaluation, the information that is attained needs to be closely examined. The performance evaluation is a tool that, if used in conjunction with a survey, can provide answers to objectives not answered on the survey.

The use of the performance evaluation, versus the survey, can be seen in this example. Students provide their impressions regarding the performance of an instructor on a survey. Can the students fairly or objectively assess the abilities of an instructor? Do students know what should and should not be taught to a class? In most cases, probably not. To attain this information, an educationally oriented evaluator needs to monitor various class sessions. The instructor(s) can be evaluated by this impartial evaluator. This information is then compared with the students' impressions.

The performance evaluation of students has already been discussed in both this chapter and Chapter 10. Both skill and written evaluations are used to assess a student's knowledge of the material. The main emphasis of this section is to look at the process used to evaluate the instructors, administration, and overall educational facilities.

INSTRUCTOR, ADMINISTRATION, AND FACILITY CHECKLISTS

Checklists are written from the main goals for a program, or they are written to reflect accepted standards of performance. Both these elements are important when developing instructor, administrative, and facility checklists. The instructor, administrative, and facility checklists are written in nearly the same format. The significant differences between them are in reference to the objectives being assessed. This difference will be illustrated through examples later in this section.

The performance evaluation for the instructor is nothing more than a modified survey. A trained evaluator is measuring the performance of an instructor against specific educational objectives. Most checklists consist of the following components:

- Basic demographic data
- Date(s) of the evaluation
- Evaluator(s) name
- Rating scale
- Specific objectives
- General comments
- Strengths/weaknesses

- Tally column
- Didactic presentation
- Skill presentation

For administration checklists, "customer-satisfaction–oriented objectives" are often used. Administration is either responsive to a customer's needs (for example, students, faculty, or the community), or there is a lack of adequate support provided to the customer. These business concepts are appropriate objectives to utilize when assessing the performance of the administration. Any educational program has bureaucratic aspects. How the paperwork is handled often impacts the quality of instruction. How can paperwork impact a program? Handouts are to be made but are forgotten. AV equipment that was to be in the classroom is missing. The classroom is too small for the size of the class. The list goes on. All these details are administrative. All impact the quality of the program. Because of their impact, administrative staff members should be assessed in the same manner that other program components are.

The administrative assessment being referred to is an overall assessment, one that is not targeted at a specific individual's performance. The assessment should focus on those administrative tasks that directly affect the classroom programs.

Translation of the Results

Let's bake a cake! A chef has flour, sugar, baking powder, salt, and so on to make the cake. These ingredients by themselves do not make the cake. The chef needs the recipe to know how much of the ingredients to use. Without the recipe, the cake is not going to turn out the way the chef wishes it to.

Translating the program evaluation information into meaningful actions is like the chef using the cake recipe. The strategy section has established the program evaluation format. Different components have been assessed throughout the program. A total program assessment has been completed. Now is the final step, assessing the assessment: Has the cake been baked correctly?

In ideal circumstances, a committee consisting of faculty, administration, and members from the community at large should review the program material. This committee will look at the areas of concern that have been identified in any of the assessments. For example, a "No" response to adequate AV materials in the classroom is a potential area of concern. Cross-checking the various surveys, for example, student opinion and instructor surveys, may provide additional support to the area of concern. In addition to negative responses, positive achievements are also reviewed. For example if a program goal was "students will achieve an 80 percent or higher on the state certification examination," and the class average was 82.4 percent, then this is a positive achievement. The people involved in the program should be given an "atta boy" for meeting this goal.

Once the committee has reviewed both the positive and negative aspects of the program, then a final report needs to be written. In this report, a summary of each assessment area is identified. Then, a discussion of the positive and negative aspects of the program is required. The report concludes with a plan of action, or program recommendations.

This plan of action specifies what parts of a program need to be changed to correct a problem or to improve the educational experience. As stated in the first section of this chapter, to have a quality program, assessment and reassessment of the program are required. This means rewriting objectives, policies, and procedures; fixing broken equipment and buying new equipment; and redefining the assessment process, so that these improvements can be assessed in the next program.

The quality improvement model is an endless circle. Only with objective input through a program assessment process can the quality of a program be improved. There are other benefits, aside from improving the program's quality, that can be gained from the program evaluation.

Summary

This chapter has looked at the approaches used to evaluate training programs and training institutes. No one evaluation tool has provided the total assessment picture. All the evaluation tools need to be evaluated before any outcome can be determined. Like any evaluation, the program evaluation is based upon educationally sound objectives and goals. These goals are placed into a strategy. Through the strategy, some are evaluated during the program. Others are evaluated after the program finishes. And yet other goals are assessed through random sampling surveys of the community served by the training institute. All provide input, so as to create an improved learning environment.

Many individuals base a training program's quality upon only single components of an evaluation, such as the written examination results. As was discussed at length, looking at only the written examination results is like looking at a tree in a forest that is a mile wide and a mile deep. Unless the whole program is objectively assessed, it is unfair to judge the creditability of a program upon only one determinant.

The key to developing a sound program evaluation, while improving the quality of the program, is to use the quality improvement circle. This approach, used in business and industry, can benefit educators. Assessing each component, at predetermined intervals allows small problems to be corrected before they become big problems. Total quality in every aspect of a training institute is the ultimate goal. A quality program leads to quality training, which leads to an improved level of performance by the graduating students. This translates into improved emergency services employees, which means a better level of service throughout the emergency service system.

Chapter 12

Internet and Computer-Based Instruction

> ➤ OBJECTIVES

- Identify the role computers have in our society.
- Identify the types of computers and computer systems that are commonly used for educational programs.
- Identify and describe the applications of the Internet.
- Describe the evolving role of technology and the use of computers.
- Define computer-assisted instruction (CAI).
- Identify the specific uses of CAI in classroom settings.
- Explore the orientation and knowledge necessary for students to use a computer.
- Examine the retention of information learned through computer-enhanced training versus traditional approaches.
- Examine how training aids have and will be affected by computerization.
- Identify hardware and software programs that are available for emergency service instructors:
    —PowerPoint
    —Computer games
    —Computer simulations
    —Computer examinations
    —CD-ROM and DVD programming
    —Computer-video interactive technology
    —Teacher-made materials
- Identify tomorrow's technology:
    —E-books
    —E-ink
    —Other forms of the Internet

Computer technology is a vital part of our daily activities, in our cars, microwaves, video games, calculators, grocery checkout counters, banking machines, Internet, e-mail, e-books, and the list goes on and on. Computers have significantly affected the emergency service industry. Just think about the equipment that relies on computers. Pagers, portable radios, handheld computers for scene reports and information, AED (automated external defibrillators), infrared thermal sensors, and CO monitors are just some of the "hardware-type" items. Software and Internet resources have changed how the emergency service industry conducts its day-to-day activities.

Emergency service classrooms, too, are computerized. Training institutes need to identify the type of computer technology that will best meet their institute's needs. Internet access, PowerPoint, and multisensory presentation equipment have changed the classroom atmosphere.

In the 1970s, few could imagine a personal computer (PC) replacing a 10-foot by 20-foot computer room. In the 1980s, only science-fiction philosophers could imagine computers, as powerful as PCs that could fit into the palm of your hand. By 1990, the possibilities of the future were realized through the expansion of the Internet. What are today's fantasies are tomorrow's reality. This chapter begins by looking at where we are today.

Computers: Pieces and Parts

Computers are a crucial part of education (Figure 12-1). Preschool, elementary, high schools/vocational schools, community colleges, and universities use computer-based technologies. College students no longer need calculators, they need personal computers, Internet access, e-mail, and an access password to their online college courses.

There are two dominant formats used in personal computers, IBM and Apple. Basic PC computer hardware consists of a computer, monitor, printer, mouse, disc drive/CD-ROM, modem/cable access card, microphone, and speakers. Computers use programs, referred to as software, to operate the computer. The software uses a variety of computer languages to tell the computer to perform specific functions.

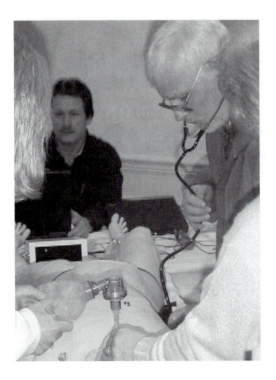

Figure 12-1
Today's computers enable realistic training opportunities for students.

Inside a computer there is an internal disc drive called the hard disc. This internal disc allows programs, photos, music, movies, and information to be stored inside the computer. Disc space is measured in bytes of digital information. Computer programs can be stored on the hard disc or onto external storage systems (i.e., CD-ROM, Zip Drives, Internet or Intranet storage systems). The term MB (megabyte), refers to the amount of hard disc space that is available to store software programs. Software programs that use digital audio and video require a lot of disc space. KB (kilobytes), MB, and GB (gigabytes) denote both a software program's size and also a storage system's maximum capacity.

The term *MB* can be misleading when "talking computers." MB also refers to another component of a computer, its RAM (random access memory). RAM is a short-term memory system that uses electronic microchips to store information needed to operate software applications. Make sure to know the RAM and hard disc memory size of a computer. If there is not enough RAM or hard disc memory, this will limit the types of software applications that can be used and stored on the computer.

How quickly a computer responds to software is determined by the size of its microprocessor. The computer within a computer is called a microprocessor or CPU. The Pentium series microprocessor is used in most IBM PC models. How quick a computer's processor is can be determined by looking at the MHz or GHz number. 450 MHz would be slower than a 1.5 GHz processor. Quickness counts, especially when using graphic-intensive software applications. This is an important aspect to keep in mind when using a software application. Check the software application for the minimum memory (RAM and hard disc) and microprocessor requirements. This information is usually found on a software application's packaging material.

Can you hear and see me? Right now you cannot since you are reading this paragraph. To see and hear software applications requires video and audio cards. These cards are actually a series of microprocessors that interpret digital audio and video signals. Three additional hardware items are required to allow a computer to see and hear, a computer monitor screen, microphone, and stereo speakers.

Today's computer monitors are brighter, sharper, clearer, and larger. Software applications that use graphic photos and images require a high picture resolution. Video streams from CD-ROMs and the Internet require even more resolution. Some monitors are not capable of handling the high-resolution demands. Larger computer monitors can cause some software applications to be distorted or not totally fit onto the screen. However, when watching movies from DVD discs, a large screen greatly improves the quality of the video image.

Multimedia stereo speakers (Figure 12-2) are needed to experience digital audio applications. The speakers can be built into a computer's monitor or can be separate units. Computer users frequently put in their favorite recording artist's CD or tune into an Internet "radio" station and listen to it while they work on their computer. Good quality speakers greatly add to a multimedia presentation. And, yes, you can get surround-sound audio systems just for your computer.

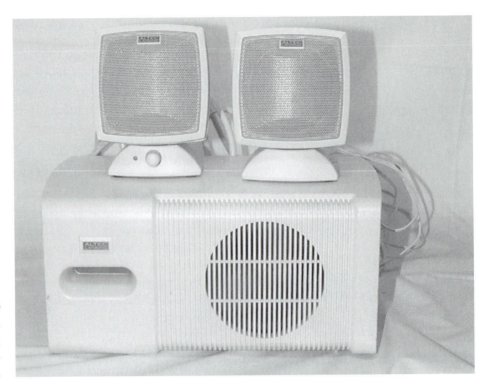

Figure 12-2
Multimedia stereo
speakers enhance a
multimedia com-
puter system.

A microphone is needed to record verbal information into a digital format. Some online chat rooms or net-meetings have audio and video capabilities. A microphone is required to communicate in these environments.

The final component is the computer's external access port. How the computer is connected to a phone or digital/cable line allows it to receive e-mail and interact with the Internet. Speed is everything when talking about the Internet. How a computer is logged onto the Internet determines how quickly it responds to Internet software applications. Getting a computer physically connected to the Internet requires hardware, software, and money.

Some of the hardware includes a dial-up modem, digital ADSL connection, satellite, or a cable-access connection. The hardware connection links a computer with a local Internet access point. The dial-up modem is the first generation of hardware connector. The minimum speed of a dial-up modem is rated at between 14K and 56K. Dial-up modems use a phone line to connect to the Internet. Dial-up modems often limit the amount of information that can be accessed quickly. This is especially true when downloading files or using some Internet applications. The result is an increased level of frustration for the computer user. Quicker access is possible using digital or cable access. Digital phone access like asymmetrical digital subscriber line (ADSL) and digital cable access allows for an almost real-time connection to the Internet. An Internet connection's speed is often determined by how much money is available.

A common misunderstanding is that the Internet is free. "Well, I do not have to pay for my e-mail and Internet access." Gaining access and using the Internet costs money to someone. Many employers or educational institutes cover the costs of their employees'/students' using the Internet. Note, there are advertising agencies that give free access if the computer user watches their clients' advertisements. Quickness costs money. The ADSL and cable access is more expensive than the dial-up modem phone access. Phone line costs plus monthly access fees are paid by someone to get and stay connected.

The last Internet component needed is the software. The software allows the hardware to connect to the Internet. AOL, Netscape, and Microsoft Explorer are examples of software browsers used to connect computers to the Internet. An Internet browser is needed to interpret information between the computer and the Internet. The next section explores what the Internet is and how these applications are used.

The Internet and How to Use It

Today's Internet grew out of computer systems that the military and military contractors used during the Cold War. Educational institutes used the Internet structure to share projects with government agencies and with each other. In 1991 the Internet was declassified. Private corporations invested money and resources into the Internet as it became known as the information superhighway.[1]

In simple terms, the Internet consists of multiple groups of computers, known as networks, which are connected together. These networks use a common computer language, such as HTML, to communicate with one another. The Internet is based on 1960s and 1970s computer technology. The computer language places limitations on what can and cannot be done on the Internet. Supplemental software has been created to operate programs outside the actual Internet environment. If an Internet site has flashy graphics and interactive programming, the site is likely using supplemental software. Insert the CD-ROM and click on "Internet Links." Go to Macromedia or Shockwave to see examples of supplemental software.

Computer and software developers, phone and cable companies, along with other investors are developing additional Internet networks. These secondary networks use sophisticated computer languages to perform tasks not possible on the traditional Internet. Real-time TV, teleconferencing, and improved software applications are just some of the improvements associated with the next generation Internet.

Whether it is the traditional Internet or the next generation Internet, the potential uses are seemingly endless. Every day, more and more users get connected and use the Internet. E-mail (electronic mail) is a frequently used Internet component. To stay in touch with someone requires a few minutes at a computer keyboard. E-mail has significantly changed how

---

[1]Lesson 2: History of the Net, www.sc.edu/bck2skol/fall/lesson2.html, Board of Trustees of the University of South Carolina, 2000; *A Brief History of the Internet*, www.isoc.org/internet/history/index.shtml, Barry M. Leiner, Vinton G. Cerf, David D. Clark, Robert E. Kahn, Leonard Kleinrock, Daniel C. Lynch, Jon Postel, Lawrence G. Roberts, Stephen Wolff, 2000.

businesses and educators communicate with clients and students. If students have questions about their assignments, their instructor likely has an e-mail address. The students can send an e-mail to ask their questions. E-mail has replaced many forms of traditional mail, which avid computer users call snail-mail. Not all correspondence is capable of being e-mailed, but more and more information is being sent via digital means.

Instead of e-mailing and waiting for a response, there are Internet applications that allow computer users to communicate with friends, family, students, coworkers, and people they do not even know. Referred to as chat rooms, electronic bulletin boards, online phone access, or net-meetings, they allow digital messages to be sent by keyboard, voice, or by video means. These forms of connection allow almost real-time access to anyone who is connected to the Internet. Information is exchanged and shared between the computer users. Many software applications allow for online sharing of programming. This enables groups of students, miles apart from one another, to simultaneously work on a project. Universities and colleges that offer online courses often use these real-time access components to communicate with their students.

Getting information about anything, anytime you need it, is a chief attribute of the Internet. Sales catalogs, businesses, libraries, government agencies, and educational institutes can be accessed via the Internet 24 hours a day. Universities and training institutes (including emergency service oriented sites) have online training programs available for personnel who do not live a nine-to-five lifestyle. College credits and continuing education credits are available from many of these Internet sites.

Information can be located on the Internet by using a search engine. These searching tools have the ability to look for specific words or phrases that are contained at an Internet site. There are multiple types of search engines. General information search engines include Yahoo, Excite, Lycos, GoTo, and AltaVista. Special search engines like Big Foot and Info-Space are used to locate people and addresses. Map Quest and Expedia.com are search engines that identify map locations, directions, and addresses. Additional engines can locate phone numbers, pictures, graphics, dictionary terms, web addresses, and the list goes on and on. A trick-of-the-trade when using a search engine is to be very specific in the topic that is being searched. Use quotation marks around terms and a plus sign between key terms to limit the search.

Assignment: Log onto the Internet. Click on one of the general search engines. Type in the words *emergency medical services*. You will likely get a lot of "hits" (responses). Now type *emergency medical services + your home state, territory, or county*. The number of hits should be reduced to a reasonable number to review.

Throughout this section, the term *Internet site* has been used. To exist on the Internet, a site must be identified by an address or location. A site listed on the World Wide Web will have a specific address called a URL (uniform resource locator).[2] An example is the Brady Publishing URL

---

[2]CenterSpan Home, www.centerspan.org, 2000.

address http://www.bradybooks.com. The first part of the address, "http://," refers to the computer language used to exchange information. The "www" refers to a site being listed on the World Wide Web. Anyone anywhere who is connected to the Internet can access the site. If a site does not have www, it may only be accessible to local network users. The next component is the site name, "bradybooks." A site name can be long or short and is followed by a three-letter suffix. The most recognized suffix is ".com." A suffix indicates the type of business, organization, or computer system the URL address is associated with. Suffixes include:

> .org = nonprofit organization
> .edu = education (college, university)
> .gov = government
> .net = local computer network
> .mil = military
> .com = commercial

Following a suffix, there maybe a backslash (/) a tilda (~) more dots (.) and other symbols and written words. These qualifiers help to specify a site location within a large Internet site. An important aspect of the address is to get each dot and backslash in the right place. Otherwise the site will not be located on the Internet. If an Internet address is known, it can be typed into the URL address line of most Internet browsers, such as AOL, Microsoft Explorer, or Netscape. Frequently used URLs can be placed into the computer's memory, which is called bookmarking the site.

Information can be printed and downloaded from the Internet. Software, such as Adobe Acrobat, allows full-page text to be printed page by page. Additional software allows text or program files, sounds, music, and pictures to be downloaded from the Internet. This is when a fast Internet connection is critical. Downloading files, especially large files, can take a long time over a slow connection.

The Internet is a valuable resource to emergency service educators and students. There are countless uses of the Internet. This section has identified general components of the Internet. Specific emergency service sites can be found on the CD-ROM. To access these sites, make sure the computer is connected to the Internet. Click on the "Emergency Services Links" on the CD-ROM.

Computer-Assisted Instruction

The buzzword in developing and using educational programming is that the programs need to be *user friendly*. A user-friendly program is one that someone who has limited or no formal computer training can easily use. Computers are a tremendous resource. Instructors should not fear the computer; rather, they should harness its power and capabilities into their presentations. Using computers should be no different than using any other audiovisual aid. The lesson material is still presented by the instructor. The computer is designed to enhance the instructor's lesson material. Let us look now at how an instructor can use the computer to enhance instructional presentations.

CAI is a catchall term that is used to describe a variety of computer-based instruction. Some programming is designed for instructor use; however, most programming is designed for student use. Computer simulations allow a student to solve real-life problems without ever leaving the classroom. Online Internet resources bring worldwide access to the latest news, techniques, and technologies. Even taking written examinations can be done using computer interactive examinations. Computer interactive laser disc programs, DVD programs, virtual reality programs, computer-interfaced manikins, satellite and compressed video systems, plus many more computer associated technologies affect emergency service classrooms.

The availability and type of computers and support equipment within a training institute become a determinant for the type of computer programming possibilities. If a training institute does not have access to personal computers, a significant monetary investment is required. To better understand the uses of CAI, the next section looks at some of the types of CAI programming available to emergency service instructors.

HARDWARE AND SOFTWARE

To implement CAI programming requires both hardware and software. Training institutes, especially universities, are investing in hardware and software resources. Computers, now more than ever, are being widely used in educational settings, including emergency services.

Instructors must know how to use computer-based resources. For example, many instructors use computers to develop lesson plans. Some training curriculums are packaged on CD-ROM. This enables an instructor to customize the lesson presentation around the needs of the students while covering the required elements of the curriculum. Also, supplemental lesson materials (puzzles, handouts, etc.), PowerPoint presentations, and quizzes are included with many textbooks. More and more materials are available on CD-ROM and on the Internet.

Let's look at some of the types of software, hardware, and resources that instructors need to know something about.

In Chapter 6, the use of PowerPoint and multimedia projectors was discussed. Additional information was provided on the CD-ROM and examples of how to use PowerPoint were identified. Through expanded digital audio and visual aids, instructors have more computer-based resources than ever. PowerPoint software allows instructors to incorporate these resources into their lesson presentations. Still images, digital video clips, and audio clips can be easily incorporated into a presentation. Instructors can do their entire presentation, including lesson plans, handouts, lecture notes, and even a quiz using a computer and a multimedia projector.

A multimedia projector can also incorporate additional computers and video components into a presentation (Figure 12-3). As noted on the CD-ROM, instructors must identify the type of multimedia system available through their training institute. Not every multimedia system has the same

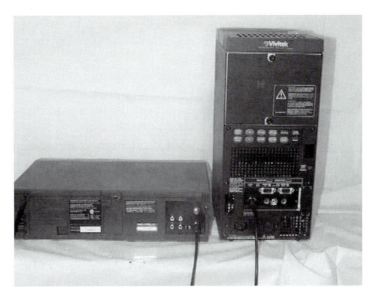

Figure 12-3
Multimedia projector.

options and capabilities. Most multimedia projectors include imports for at least one computer and a video system. Video can be imported from a DVD, videotape, or cable-TV system. By depressing a button on the projector or its remote, an instructor can switch between a PowerPoint presentation and a video import.

As a reminder, make sure to keep a balance between going too high tech and assuring the best interests of a presentation. Balance the presentation with the reality of what resources exist within a training institute.

COMPUTER-BASED EXAMINATIONS

Throw away the no. 2 pencils if an instructor is using a computer-based examination. An entire written test can be taken on a computer. Students log onto the examination program. A series of computer screens takes the student from question 1 through question 100 and then back and forth among the questions as required. When the student is finished, the computer tabulates the score, and the student can immediately see the results. At the same time, the computer records the examination score in a computer file for the instructor to reference after all the students have completed the examination.

Multiple options and enhancements can be incorporated into the examination format. For initial learning, the computer examination can be modified to a tutorial mode. When a student incorrectly answers a question, the computer shows the student a passage that contains the correct answer. For learning disabled students, the examination can be orally read to the students via headphones. This enables the students to see and hear the questions and answers. This enhancement provides capable disabled learners with an avenue for success instead of frustration. Other exam possibilities include the use of animations. A heart can be shown pumping or a power hydraulic tool spreading a door open. Further enhancements include digitizing photographs and video clips. A digitized image is a photograph that is converted electronically so that the computer can identify it. Digital photographs can be used as background images for an examination question.

How does an instructor make computer examinations? Commercial software authoring programs are available for an instructor with limited computer experience to put together a computer-based examination. Many programs allow the text of a question to be changed without erasing the background or other graphic material. Thus an examination question can be changed fairly easily. More sophisticated examination programs (e.g., animations, digitally enhanced photos, tutorials) do require an instructor to have more than just a casual knowledge of examination construction. The end product is a highly professional examination that is designed for a specific lesson plan.

Incorporated into most computer examinations is a random question selection process. Examination questions are pulled from a bank of questions and are randomly assigned to each student. Students can be sitting side by side and will be answering completely different questions. This provides a unique form of test security, rarely available with written examinations.

As powerful as computer examinations are, there are limitations. These include cost, computer access, and test security. To effectively use these exams students need to have access to a computer. As commonplace as computers seem to be, many emergency service classrooms do not have computer access to computer labs. There needs to be enough computers for an entire class to use. If there is not sufficient computer access for the students, the use of computerized testing may need to be reevaluated. Yes, these examinations can be taken online. Any exam, especially a computer examination, is not to be a cooperative effort between students. The identity of the person sitting at an online computer terminal cannot be easily assured. Consequently, before developing a CAI examination, look at these limitations and assure they are addressed.

COMPUTER-BASED TEXTBOOKS/SOFTWARE

Instead of reading this textbook in a paper format, it could be viewed on a computer or on a handheld notepad known as an e-book (Figure 12-4). Colorful graphic images, coupled with clearly written text, make this an innovative computer-based learning approach. The e-book notepad is capable of holding several complete textbooks. Textbooks, novels, newspapers, or magazines can be downloaded into the e-book. Full time students will enjoy one of the advantages of the e-book, a lighter weight to their book bag.

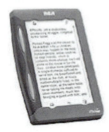

Figure 12-4
E-books can be contained within a small hand-held unit. Books are downloaded into the e-book.

All the textbooks needed for a semester can be stored within the palm-held e-book. RCA is the principle manufacturer of the e-book, and Gemstar is the software vendor for e-book.[3] The e-book is slowly making its way onto colleges campuses. Textbook manufacturers are converting paper-based textbooks into the digital e-book format. Disadvantages to the e-book include a lack of a printed copy, cost of acquiring the e-Book, and copyright issues. Once accustomed to using the e-book, users tend to prefer it to their printed textbook counterparts. Insert the CD-ROM and click on the e-book button for additional information.

COMPUTERIZED TUTORIAL PROGRAMS

A tutorial program is a combination of written material, high-quality graphic pictures, and an oral narrative. Every two to three pages, a series of two or three questions is asked. If a student answers them correctly, the computer acknowledges the student with an "atta boy" on the screen. If the student misses a question, the computer returns to the point in the text where the answer is highlighted. The student rereads this section and the program continues. At the next question section, the question that was previously missed is asked again. If instructors can make their own tutorial programs, this personalization becomes an important teaching adjunct.

Tutorial programs usually offer a student several presentation formats. One format is a written text without oral enhancements. Another option is to have specific words enhanced. These are called *hot words*. This allows the student to hear the pronunciation of a word and then to see/hear the definition of the word. The final option is to have the entire written text orally read to the student. The graphic and text screens usually remain the same for each option. Most tutorial presentations start with a visual or oral introduction of the program and then provide directions for the use of the program.

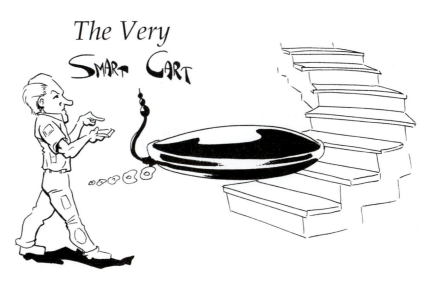

EMTs in tomorrow's EMS world may not even have to worry about lifting patients up a set of stairs. The "Very Smart Cart" will fly the patient up the stairs and into the ambulance.

---

[3]Interview with Johanna Schmid, Gemstar, December 2000.

Being able to digitize photographs enhances the basic tutorial program. Photographs of accident scenes, pieces of equipment, or images of injuries can be incorporated into text screens. These images have amazing detail and look like an actual still photograph. Digital photos usually do not require additional hardware to be displayed. However, they do take up computer memory, so make sure that the computer has sufficient memory.

Commercial tutorial programming does exist. These tutorial programs need to be closely reviewed by an instructor. If a program contains material that does not meet the lesson's objectives, it should not be used. Computer programs are no different from any other teaching adjunct.

Tutorial programs can be motivational learning tools for students. But some students want to have more interaction and less text material. For these students, there is the review program.

REVIEW PROGRAM

The review program, often called the drill-and-practice program, is a program that provides a student with a series of questions and text screens. The content of the program is centered on asking the student probing questions and providing help screens when a student responds inappropriately to a question. These types of programs are excellent for students who want to refresh their knowledge of a subject. They are also ideal for examination preparation. These programs are not examinations per se, but because they are a learning tool, they fall into the review category.

Computer graphics and digital images improve the quality of these programs. Instructors may wish to use these programs with students who have a good knowledge of the material and do not need visual or oral assistance. Once these students use the review program, they are probably ready for the next two types of programs, simulations and computer games.

SIMULATIONS

You and your crew respond to a reported stabbing in the alley next to the BP Bar. Police are on the scene, and the scene is safe. You find a male, about 20 to 25 years old. He is supine, rolling side to side, obviously in distress, has a blood-soaked shirt and pants. Which of the following options might be your first actions?

1. Perform a primary survey
2. Implement appropriate universal precautions
3. Conduct a head-to-toe survey
4. Request a backup

This is a narrative example of a simulation program. An enhanced simulation includes pictures and diagrams that enhance this narrative description. The narrative could be an EMS, fire, or rescue simulation. As the student answers questions, the computer revises the situation. Appropriate actions improve the situation, while inappropriate actions worsen the situation.

With just a narrative format—that is, with no other enhancements—students can interact with the computer to solve the situation. In the initial example, the situation was EMS related. But there are simulations that are fire related. Students are given a structure-fire scenario and must position their resources to control the fire. Just as when a patient's condition worsens when improper care is given, the fire progresses and can involve other nearby structures.

A simulation allows students to explore and problem solve realistic situations. Instructors strive to have students function at the upper levels of the knowledge taxonomy. Using a computer simulation is one way to encourage high levels of comprehension, while having fun doing it.

Included on the CD-ROM are two examples of computer-based simulations. Brady Publishing MERS (Medical Emergency Response Simulator) places a student into various situations to which they must react. The second simulation example is an Internet link to the Brady Internet site, www.bradybooks.com. At this site you can select from different case studies. Use the interactive features in both simulation examples.

COMPUTER GAMES

Using computer games is an enhancement of the simulation concept. What is the difference? The difference is that there is a competitive aspect. Points are awarded for successful performance. A student plays to beat another student's score. Or a student tries to beat the clock, before it is too late to save the patient or building. In this concept, points are deducted (e.g., the clock ticks down). If the right steps are not taken, large chunks of time are deducted. When correct procedures are initiated, no deductions occur. Competition adds to the motivation level. The educational value is improved and the students are able to interact. They are doing something with their knowledge.

Computer games should be used prudently by instructors. Not every session or subject is suited for a computer game. Moreover, commercially made games are relatively scarce. By far, there are many more simulations and review programs than there are computer games. The trend is clear, though; computer games will become more readily available for emergency service instructors.

As with other forms of educational programming, simulations and games need to be reviewed for their content. Many programs may not be suited for an instructor's lesson plan. In addition, the cost and availability of the programs and the availability of computers may inhibit the use of these programs.

A completely new level of simulation and learning is now possible with the use of the digital programming and laser disc interactive programming. The next section reviews this exciting area of computer aided instruction.

DIGITIZED PROGRAMMING

Programs now available on CDs have stereo-quality sound and high-quality graphics married with text screens. These programs range from digitized "animated photos" that make photos appear to be in motion to full-motion video clips. Instead of looking at a diagram of an accident scene or only reading a narrative description, by using digital technology, an actual series of accident scene photos can be displayed in full color. The CD programs can have an oral narration and background music or realistic sounds, which create a realistic program on the computer screen or multimedia projector.

The student has control of the program. As a program progresses, it asks questions for the student to answer. Many programs offer special information functions. For example, if a student wanted to know more about the power hydraulic gasoline power unit, there could be a series of digital photos and oral narration that would explain the power unit. For students who do not need to know any further information, the main program keeps operating.

Digital programs are commercially made and designed for a national audience. Caution and review are prerequisites that an instructor must employ when using these programs. In comparison to the laser programs, CD programs tend to be less expensive. They are not full-motion programs, but they are close enough to be in the same neighborhood.

COMPUTER INTERACTIVE LASER-DISC PROGRAMS

A computer interactive laser disc brings full-motion video to the fingertips of a student. Instead of viewing still photos, graphic images, text screens, or drawings, students sit in front of a "computer television." With most television programs, you cannot control the action. With a computer laser-disc interactive program, however, the student controls everything, all with the touch of a mouse button or a touch-screen monitor.

The laser discs used for most systems are commercially made and are designed for a national audience. Some states, Idaho, in particular, have been using this technology and have produced their own laser disc programming. This has enabled Idaho to make specific programming to fit the state's training needs.[4]

The cost of a learning station runs from $6,000 and up. Commercially made laser discs start at $450 and up. If you are interested in making your own laser disc, plan on spending over $100,000 to produce it. Clearly, the start-up costs for a learning station are significant. Laser discs are not cheap, especially if you make your own. So why invest and use this technology? This question has been posed and answered by *Fortune* 500 companies, the military, and numerous universities. There is not one answer, but many answers. Let's look at some of the more persuasive answers that have been identified in various journals and reports.

> Robert S. Porter conducted a CAI training program for paramedics in the state of Michigan who were participating in a continuing education program. Lecture, video tapes, and CAI were evaluated for their

---

[4]Paul B. Anderson et al., "Interactive Technology: EMS Training Goes Online in Idaho," *Journal of Emergency Medical Services,* October 1990.

effectiveness. A pretest, posttest, and a 60-day posttest were administered. For the posttest and the 60-day posttest, the CAI-trained paramedics retained more information than those taught by lecture and video tapes.[5]

British Telecom needed to train 6,000 managers within an 18-month time period. Traditional teaching approaches made this type of training cost prohibitive. IVD was selected and saved the corporation over $2 million.[6]

The *Videodisc Monitor* reported in January 1990 that Xerox, Ford Motor Company, and Federal Express were impressed with the time savings, coupled with the cost savings, that their IVD systems provided to their companies. Increased retention and recall of information were noted by the training directors from these corporations.[7]

In a presentation paper, Ann L. Lyness identified the results from a study that compared IVD training with traditional CPR training. Two randomized groups of students were selected. The results indicated a statistical significance for IVD training in a conscious airway obstruction, becomes unconscious airway obstruction, and unconscious airway obstruction. In other component areas, such as one-rescuer CPR, two-rescuer CPR, infant CPR, infant conscious airway obstruction, and infant unconscious airway obstruction there were no statistical significances noted.[8]

In her doctoral dissertation, Mary E. Aukerman presented similar findings to those noted by Ann Lyness. Registered nurses were taught using the IVD CPR training and the traditional CPR approach. She noted in her conclusion that there were no statistical significances between the two approaches. She did note that the RNs preferred the IVD approach and that a significant reduction in instructor time was noted. She noted that IVD is equally effective as the traditional CPR approach, plus it is more cost effective and a preferred method of instruction.[9]

These five abstracts identify some of the many research studies that have been done with IVD training. IVD training is as good as, or better than, traditional training approaches. A reduction in instructor training time is noted, mainly because students can use the system at their own pace. Retention and extended retention of information appear to be improved over traditional methods. Students appear to like the IVD training, based on

---

[5]Robert S. Porter, "Efficacy of Computer-Assisted Instruction in the Continuing Education of Paramedics," *Annals of Emergency Medicine* 4 (1991), pp. 380–384.

[6]"BT Cost Saving for Appraisal and Counselling Training," *The Videodisc Monitor*, 1990.

[7]"Effectiveness of Using Interactive Technologies for Training," *The Videodisc Monitor*, January 1990.

[8]Ann L. Lyness, "Effectiveness of Interactive Video to Teach CPR Theory and Skills," research paper presentation to Association for Educational Communications and Technology, January 1985.

[9]Mary Elizabeth Aukerman, "Effectiveness of an Interactive Video Approach for CPR Recertification of Registered Nurses," doctoral dissertation, University of Pittsburgh, 1986.

postevaluation studies. There are appreciable start-up costs. Major corporations have noted that even with these high initial costs, in the long term there will be a significant return on their investment. Thus IVD may be a worthwhile investment for instructors and training institutes to consider in the context of a long term investment.

Computerized Training Equipment

Training programs have already been using computer-enhanced training manikins and equipment for some time. Computers control more and more field equipment. Medical training programs have seen probably the largest use of computer technology, but fire and rescue training programs are not far behind (Figure 12-5).

Training equipment should reflect the equipment that is being used by field personnel. Even training manikins should be realistic and accurately report a student's performance. The computer chip, used in training and field equipment, has begun another historic change in how field personnel perform their jobs.

Medical training equipment such as CPR manikins, ECG dysrhythmia generators, defibrillators, automated external defibrillators, external pacing units, automatic BP and pulse monitors, pulse oximeters, and end-tidal CO_2 monitors are acquiring more and more computer enhancements.

Fire and rescue training and field equipment have been enhanced by computer technology. Some equipment includes computerized pump panels, motion detector devices, hazardous material monitors, thermal

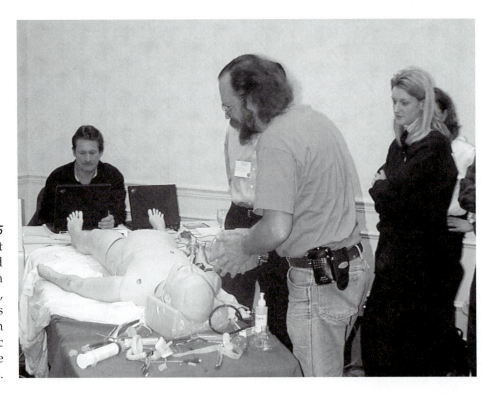

Figure 12-5
Students interact with a computerized manikin that has a pulse, respiration, and heartbeat. This almost real manikin creates a realistic learning experience for students.

detection units, atmospheric monitors, and specialized communication equipment for use with SCBA systems.

Where is educational equipment heading? The path is set for more and more equipment to become computer enhanced. Instructors will need to become computer literate because the trend is set in the direction for further computer use in the years to come. So what can instructors look forward to seeing and using? The next section looks at the future classroom technologies, which will become the standard of instruction.

A Look at Advanced Technologies

Not using too much clairvoyance, the following technologies will likely impact tomorrow's classroom. These technologies may have already been incorporated into some classrooms and will likely gain further prominence.

VIRTUAL REALITY

Virtual reality is an awesome computer concept. The applicability, coupled with the potential uses of this technology, are endless. Besides being an awesome video-game format, what is virtual reality?[10]

Through the use of computer-created images, an individual is taken into realistic situations without leaving a room. Full-motion computer images coupled with digital sound and a variety of computer sensors are used to create real-life experiences and situations. Military or commercial airline flight simulators are frequently used as a starting point for a comparison to the virtual reality experience. But virtual reality is much more than that.

The hardware of the virtual reality system enables a person to feel and become an active participant in the computer simulation. Most systems consist of a closed helmet, which is positioned over the eyes and allows the wearer to see only the images displayed on small stereoscopic screens. Stereo headphones provide the digital sounds. With special sensors positioned onto the individual's hands, torso, and legs, the virtual reality system allows a person to escape from reality into a computer-generated environment.

Individuals, once in the simulation, can control their movements in the simulation. The hand sensors permit objects to be picked up and moved around in the virtual world. Leg sensors allow a person to walk through the simulation. Once in the virtual world, a person becomes a part of the simulation.

Real-world applications are endless. Japanese, British, and U.S. companies are using this technology in a variety of fields. From walking prospective homeowners through a floor plan to providing teenagers with the ultimate computer-game experience, virtual reality programming is being produced.

---

[10]This section is based on the following articles in *NewMedia Journal,* January 1990: Tony Reveaux, "Virtual Reality Gets Real"; Gaye L. Graves, "NASA's Virtual Reality" and "Invasion of the Digital Puppets."

What can emergency service instructors expect to attain from virtual reality systems? It very well could turn the present-day educational process upside down. EMS students could pick up defibrillator paddles and defibrillate virtual reality patients. Firefighters can hold simulated hose lines and battle a virtual reality fire. Rescue students can rappel off a virtual reality cliff and rescue an injured hiker. Students will be able to experience real-life events before they actually occur. Virtual reality can be a tremendous resource and teaching tool for instructors.

The cost of a virtual reality system is considerable. As with other technologies, in time, the systems will become more affordable. However, if there is an emerging technology that instructors should watch, it is virtual reality.

HIGH-DEFINITION TELEVISION

A key element in the expansion of computerizing classrooms will be to provide monitors that display realistic images. HDTV is dramatically improving the quality of the picture shown on television monitors.[11] HDTV uses digital information to display the enhanced pictures. Television sets use vertical lines to display an image. On a standard television set there are about 480 resolution lines, compared to HDTV, which has 2,000 resolution lines. The pictures shown on HDTV appear as clear as a photograph. The HDTV receives digital information from fiber-optic telephone lines. Through the use of digital transmission, an increased amount of information can be shown in addition to the television images.

The potential for HDTV is unlimited. Currently, HDTV is enhancing computer-graphic images, especially for graphic images known as holograms. These are 3-D images that require a high-resolution screen to provide adequate detail. Additionally, HDTV monitors are already being used to enhance computer networks in major corporations. Linked via a fiber-optic telephone network, two-way audio and visual transmission of information is possible. Normal television and computer monitors cannot handle the increased data that computer networks require. The HDTV is designed to handle this increased volume of information and provides an improved visual image.

FLAT-SCREEN TV

Going along with the HDTV is the larger flat-screen television. Flat-screen televisions come in sizes ranging from 16-inch screens to 52-inch screens. The flat screen uses a plasma base, which is electronically charged. The picture quality is equal to real-life environments. The realistic quality cannot be matched by traditional television sets.

Flat-screen television can support a variety of formats. DVD, video, HDTV, and computer inputs can be used on the flat screen. A separate tuner

---

[11]This section is based on Nicholas P. Negroponte, "Products and Services for Computer Networks," *Scientific American*, September 1991.

source is often required. Augmenting the flat screen are equally impressive audio surround-sound systems. The sensory experience is awesome when the two systems are combined.

The price of flat-screen systems ranges from $1,000 to $20,000. Clearly they are not for everyone's budget. As with most technologies, look for prices to lower and more features to be included on newer models.

COMPUTER SCRATCH PADS AND LIVE BOARDS

"Throw away the pens, pencils, chalk, and dry-image pens" will be the standard approach when scratch pads and live boards become the norm.[12] A scratch pad is a computer display screen that reads information that is written directly onto it via an electronic pen. These pads are flat screens that are about 12 inches by 12 inches by 2 inches. A live board is a larger screen, 3 feet by 4 feet. Both can be linked together, or they can be used independently.

Instead of using paper, students can use a scratch pad to take notes or prepare information. When linked together, the instructor and the students will be able to see the information at the same time. People will be able to write comments directly onto their screens, and they will be transmitted throughout the other boards.

Using the larger live boards with several scratch boards, an instructor and students will be able to discuss openly any information that is displayed. Using an electronic pen, the instructor can write onto the live board and have the same information appear on everyone's scratch pads. Memory chips will be able to retain the information that is discussed, and it can be downloaded to make a hard copy.

COMPUTER NETWORKS

Already introduced, classroom networks can greatly improve the information exchange between an instructor and the students. But there is a much larger potential use for the HDTV, scratch pads, and live boards. Instead of a single class being networked, the potential exists for multiple classrooms to be linked together.[13] One instructor could instruct hundreds of students at the same time. All the students could be interlinked and could communicate from either their scratch pads or live boards.

These networks need to be fiber-optically or satellite linked. The state of Virginia, for example, is now using satellite transmissions to deliver TV presentations to rural EMS providers.[14] With a satellite system already in place, enhancing it to use a computer network is a consideration for the future. Students in a rural classroom could use computer scratch pads to communicate with a larger class of students in an urban classroom.

---

[12]This section is based on Mark Weiser, "The Computer for the Twenty-First Century," *Scientific American*, September 1991.

[13]This section is based on Michael Dertouzos, "Communications, Computers, and Networks," *Scientific American*, September 1991.

[14]Ibid.

The potential and variety of uses for these computer networks are endless. There is a tremendous initial investment that is required to attain the necessary hardware and software. As technological advancements continue, these initial costs will be lessened. The need for quality information will make these computer systems the norm for classrooms in the future.

E-INK: TOMORROW'S PAPERLESS SOLUTION

Already mentioned is the e-book. It uses a notepad computer that allows a user to view text and graphics. Another technology in its early development has endless possibilities. It is call e-ink. E-ink is quite different from the e-book. E-ink uses a flexible thin display. Electric charges, positive and negative, are passed through individual cells that change color. The result is the ability to have the display change shapes and form different letters.

The exact mechanics of how the final product will look are unknown. Presently the display is rolled and placed inside a tube. The text is changed each time it is slid in and out of the tube. As with e-books, newspapers, magazines, novels, and textbooks can be downloaded into the e-ink display. With the flexible display, reading from the display is similar to reading from a newspaper.

Other applications can be found in communication systems and advertising venues. For example, an advertising executive in New York could electronically change an 8-foot wide e-ink advertising board located along a highway in California.

E-ink and e-books are alternatives to becoming a paperless society. Instead of reading a newspaper printed on paper, you may be reading it on an e-book or e-ink display. Go to the CD-ROM and click on the e-ink link to learn more about this evolving technology.

Summary

Since the 1970s, there has been a tremendous explosion of computer technology. There are now palm-size computers that do as much or more than a roomful of computers did in the past. Computers are a part of most peoples' daily lives. The trend is clear, computers will become more powerful and will be available to the general population.

The Internet has changed how students and instructors learn and explore information. Instructors who underutilize computer resources will likely be less effective in tomorrow's classrooms. More and more emphasis is toward computers and technology in all phases of emergency service education.

With virtual-reality software and hardware development, traditional practice sessions will be accomplished without even touching an actual piece of equipment. The information exchange between students and instructors, in multiple training sites, will become a real possibility.

Even today's computer programming, such as computer simulations and games, are a quantum leap ahead of many traditional teaching concepts. Instructors need to use their present-day knowledge, but they also need to expand their thoughts into probing the future of computer-enhanced instruction. Tomorrow's classrooms will not have fewer computers, they will have more. Instructors who are computer illiterate need to gain computer literacy, because tomorrow's classroom will demand it.

Chapter 13

Realism Concepts

➤ **OBJECTIVES**

- Discuss the role of realism in classrooms.
- Identify the various ways to introduce realism in a lesson.
- Review the creation and use of scenarios in classroom settings.
- Define the terms *makeup* and *moulage.*
- Identify types of simulation supplies.
- Address the role of props and facilities.
- Identify the importance of acting out the scenario by the actors.
- Identify and describe injuries and emergency conditions that can be effectively simulated:
  —Shocklike appearance
  —Abrasions
  —Burns
  —Sucking chest wound
  —Lacerations
  —Fractures
  —Amputations
  —Bruise
- Identify when and where to use realism concepts.

In the previous chapter, computers were identified as being a source for providing realism. There are many ways to incorporate realism into a presentation. This chapter addresses realism concepts that can be used in emergency service presentations. (Figure 13-1).

When realism is mentioned, thoughts of grease pencils and fake blood are conjured up. This is only one aspect of realism. Realistic concepts are much more involved than just dumping fake blood onto a simulated patient. Emergency service environments are themselves realistic settings. Burn buildings, cliffs and hillsides, firefighting apparatus, training equipment, or even lab specimens are realistic. An instructor needs only to look within the classroom to identify equipment and concepts to use.

Realism concepts are based upon the lesson plan. The realism that is used must fit the lesson's material. To begin, the when, where, and how questions about creating realism concepts need to be identified. Then specific realism concepts are identified, including the use of makeup and moulage techniques. The CD-ROM contains additional examples of photos depicting injuries, settings, and creation techniques. Insert the CD-ROM and click on "Realism."

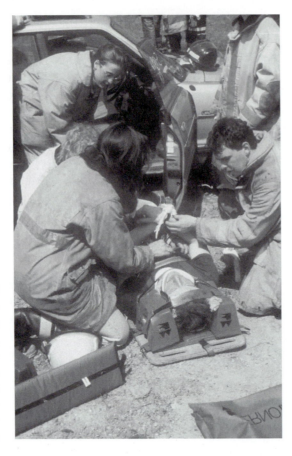

Figure 13-1
Instead of just pretending that a patient is severely injured, students can participate in a simulation, which provides them with a realistic situation and a realistic-looking patient.

Realism's Role

Adult learners need to have realism to have an effective learning experience.[1] Thus, realistic concepts should be a part of every lesson presentation. Providing actual contact with realistic looking situations helps prepare students for real-life experiences. An instructor's role, then, is to use realistic equipment, situations, and course materials that simulate real-life settings. The role of realism is to bring the real-life situations into a controlled learning environment.

Simulation Facilities

Some training institutes are fortunate to have simulation facilities. Buildings such as smokehouses, burn buildings, rappelling towers, hazardous material pits, propane fire simulators, and driving simulation rooms are some of the types of facilities that are available to many emergency-service classes. Community colleges, state fire fighting academies, and even local service agencies, such as power companies, have these types of facilities.

---

[1]This discussion relies on Malcolm Knowles, *The Adult Learner: A Neglected Species* (Houston, Tex.: Gulf, 1990).

However, when instructors do not have access to a permanent simulation facility, they must look for a next best choice. Instructors who use facilities that are not intended for a specific use, like a burn building, must be very safety conscious. A full safety check of the structure must be done. This includes making additional exits from the structure, placing ventilation holes in the roof, positioning escape ladders at the second-floor windows, having interior safety crews in the building at all times, identifying a secondary water supply source, and having separate fire suppression equipment from that being used in the training activity. All of the instructors need to be acutely aware of the potential dangers when using an off-site learning environment. Realism is one thing, but getting students injured is another issue completely.

For medical training programs and vehicle rescue courses, automobiles, trucks, or buses are used. These too need to be free of potential hazards. Gas tanks and other flammable liquids should be removed from the vehicles. Vehicles placed on their sides should be stabilized before a patient actor is placed inside. Fully charged hand lines and backup rescue crews and equipment should be ready in case there is a problem during a training session.

When using any uncontrolled simulation facility, such as wrecked vehicles, an instructor must be able to anticipate, and attempt to prevent, a hazardous situation from developing. A safety officer should be identified to observe the overall activities. Safety is the number one concern; then comes the realism.

Realism Tools

Emergency service instructors have a wealth of equipment and resources to use as realism tools. The training equipment itself is a realistic learning aid. There are some lesson presentations that, by their nature, are excellent settings for realism.

Let's consider human anatomy. Students could review charts, diagrams, or interact with a computer-based anatomy simulation. But being able to see and touch actual lab specimens takes on a completely different level of realism. Depending on a training institute's resources, conducting an actual cadaver lab could be an invaluable resource. This kind of realism leaves a lasting impression on the students.

Another example is to tap into resources available within the community—for instance, contacting the electric company for a hands-on demonstration of handling downed power lines. Many power companies have prevention programs as part of their community outreach. Showing students the actual equipment and talking to the people who handle live power lines every day is a more realistic approach to teaching an electrical hazards presentation.

The resources for creating realism are within every instructor's reach. All instructors need to do is to spend a little time to identify how they can use realism in their lesson presentation.

SCENARIOS

Before placing a patient actor inside an overturned vehicle, there needs to be a written guideline to use for setting up a realistic setting. A scenario helps to make sure everyone behind the scene knows what to expect. This means that the safety officer, backup rescue personnel, and assistant instructors all need to know what to expect. A scenario allows them to anticipate the actions of the students and to provide a safe rescue simulation.

When the lesson plan is being written, the scenarios should be written. An instructor identifies the equipment and resources needed for the simulation. Even indoor classroom sessions should use predeveloped scenarios. The scenario identifies the actions for the instructor, the students, and the patient actors.

To make a scenario real, several components are needed. One component has already been discussed, that being the use of on-site and off-site training facilities. There are other components, such as selecting and using patient actors, effective makeup concepts, and props that make the situation appear to be real. Any of these components can affect how realistic a presentation becomes for the students.

MAKEUP AND MOULAGE

These two terms are often used together, but they do have different meanings. Makeup is the use of a cosmetic type of product. Moulage refers to molds, plastics, or rubber styled injuries. Used together, creating realistic-looking injuries is not a problem (Figure 13-2).

Moulage products have gotten a bad rap for looking fake. But when they are used with cosmetic products, they can look very realistic. It is all in how an instructor uses the products. Makeup looks fake and inappro-

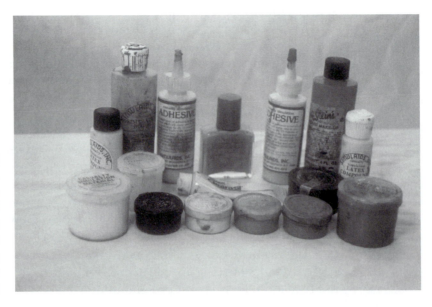

Figure 13-2
Shown here are a variety of makeup supplies. These and additional supplies are used to create realistic-looking injuries. (*Photo by Richard Gibbons, Jr.*)

priate when too much is applied. A general rule of thumb is the least is the best. Having patient actors looking like Smurfs or clowns is not the appropriate use of these products.

There are a vast number of makeup and moulage products that can be used to simulate injuries. The following list identifies some of the products that are available:

- Grease liners (white, blue, red, yellow, brown, black, natural)
- Compact/base foundation
- Red fingernail polish
- Latex adhesive
- Glycerin
- Cotton balls/tissue paper
- Plexiglas
- Alka-Seltzer tablets
- Amputation moulage
- Evisceration moulage
- Fresh rack-of-ribs
- Scissors
- Wooden/plastic tongue blade and so on
- Eyeliner (blue and red)
- Mortician's wax
- Coagulated blood
- Ashes/charcoal/dirt
- Vaseline/cosmetic mask
- Simulated bones
- Bleeding wounds/bleeding bags
- Laceration moulage
- Fresh link sausage
- Cold cream
- Plasteline
- Latex gel effects
- Q-tips, stipple sponges, combs, etc.

A variety of wounds can be made with these products. There are common injuries or conditions that instructors simulate quite frequently. Those include a shocklike appearance, lacerations, abrasions, bruises, fractures, burns, amputations, and sucking chest wounds. If an instructor can become proficient at using these eight simulations, most other simulations will be created without a lot of difficulty. The best advice when using makeup products is to be conservative in the application of makeup. Too little can be corrected, too much usually cannot be easily corrected. Let's look at how to apply these eight types of makeup and moulage.

Safety Note: Before applying any makeup or moulage products to a patient actor, ask the actor if he is allergic to cosmetic-based or latex products. Many of these products can be irritants, and the last thing an instructor needs to have is a true anaphylactic shock condition in the patient actor. Also, tell students participating in the session that the simulated victims have been made up with cosmetic and latex products.

When it is possible, before applying makeup to a patient actor have the actor apply a very thin coating of cold cream to the areas that will be made up. This helps the actor to clean up after the simulations are completed (Figure 13-3).

Shocklike Appearance

Both medical emergency and trauma patients experience poor tissue perfusion. A patient's skin color becomes pale, and in severe cases the skin appears gray or bluish (Figure 13-4). The skin is usually cool and is sweaty. Keeping these signs of shock in mind, now comes the process of simulating a patient with a shocklike condition.

Apply a thin coating of grease, powder, or other make-up product onto a patient actor's face, ears, neck, hands, arms, and legs. Any body part that

Figure 13-3
The patient-actor applies a thin coating of cold cream onto the exposed skin prior to applying makeup. This allows for easy removal of the makeup following the simulation. (*Photo by Richard Gibbons, Jr.*)

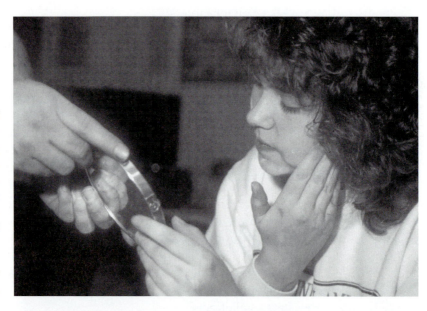

Figure 13-4
The instructor blends in the blue liner to create the "greyish" appearance. (*Photo by Richard Gibbons, Jr.*)

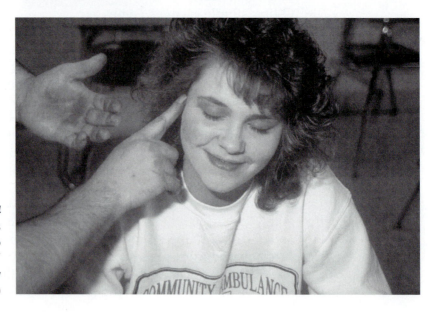

is immediately exposed or will be exposed during an assessment needs to be made up. This thin coating should be blended into the patient's skin, so that there are no obvious blobs or streaks. If using blue-based makeup, use only a very small amount of blue and carefully blend it into the base makeup. Blue coloring is a powerful color and many patient actors end up looking like Smurfs instead of patients in a shocklike state.

To finish off the shocklike appearance, use either a water bottle with a spray button or glycerin (Figure 13-5). Apply either product onto the exposed body surfaces. Be careful to avoid spraying these products in an actor's eyes, nose, ears, or mouth.

With the shocklike appearance completed, other injuries can be added. The glycerin or water should be applied only after additional injuries have been applied.

Lacerations

There are many ways to apply makeup and moulage to simulate lacerations (Figure 13-6). The commonly used approaches include plasteline, mortician's wax latex, or small plastic moulage wounds.

Using the plasteline or mortician's wax allows additional injuries to be added to a basic laceration (Figure 13-7). These can include Plexiglas, bleeding lines, even bone fragments. Note, male patient actors with hairy arms, legs, chest, or back may not be the best choice for lacerations. One of the first applications to the site is a thin coating of latex glue. The latex needs to dry. The latex tends to hold the wax onto the skin, especially when dressings are being applied repeatedly to the area.

Depending on how big the laceration will be, take a walnut-size amount of the plasteline or wax and roll it around in your hands. This tends to soften it and allows for a smoother application. Flatten it out and apply it onto the site. Using a wooden tongue blade or an artist's knife, smooth it out evenly onto the site (Figure 13-8). After this is done, take the edge of the

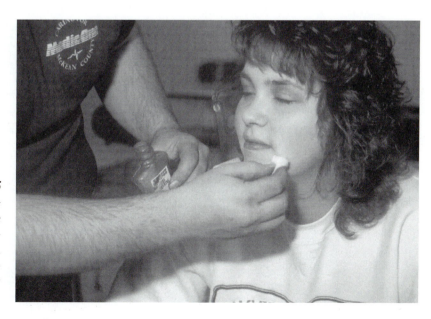

Figure 13-5
To finish the shock-like appearance, the instructor uses glycerin to simulate a sweaty texture to the skin. (*Photo by Richard Gibbons, Jr.*)

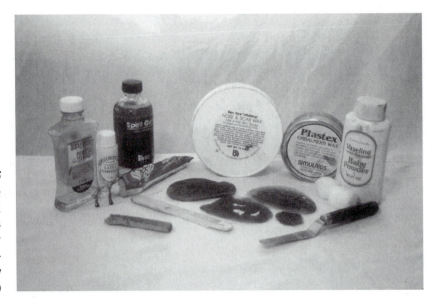

Figure 13-6
Shown here are the makeup and moulage supplies that are commonly used to simulate lacerations. (*Photo by Richard Gibbons, Jr.*)

blade and draw a jagged line to simulate the laceration site (Figure 13-9). It may be necessary to heighten the laceration by making a lip along the edge of the laceration. Using the natural color grease liner or cosmetic foundation, apply a color that closely matches the patient actor's skin color. When using plasteline, brown or dark brown colored plasteline can be added. Blend the colors together until it matches the patient actor's skin color. To add color to the laceration, use red liner, red fingernail polish, or warmed red latex gel in the line that is cut into the wax (Figure 13-10).

The last component to apply is the coagulated blood in the wound. It is important to apply the blood only when the patient actor is lying in the position for the scenario. Apply small amounts of blood into the laceration. Gravity will do the rest. After each group of students, the blood will need

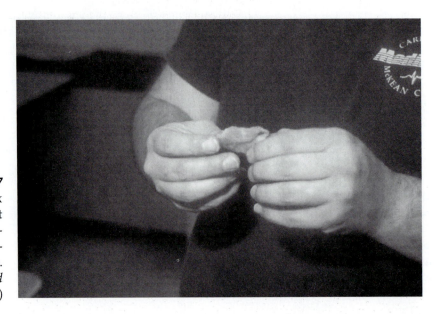

Figure 13-7
The mortician's wax is easier to apply if it is molded by the instructor prior to applying it to the site. (*Photo by Richard Gibbons, Jr.*)

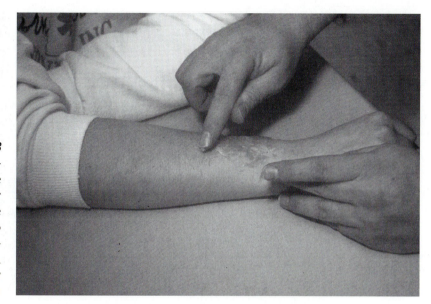

Figure 13-8
Once the wax is applied, it needs to be smoothed out. For the final touch, use an artist's knife to smooth out any remaining rough edges. (*Photo by Richard Gibbons, Jr.*)

to be reapplied. When using the warmed red latex gel, rarely does a lot of blood need to be reapplied.

Easily added to the laceration are either bone fragments or Plexiglas. Once the laceration has been made, the bones or Plexiglas can be inserted (Figure 13-11). The laceration lip can be pushed into the bones or Plexiglas to hold them in place. Red grease liner, fingernail polish, or warmed red latex gel can be added to both the laceration and to the bones or Plexiglas fragments. Caution needs to be used, so a real laceration does not occur. Be sure to have enough plasteline or wax around the objects to hold them in place.

Just as in the basic laceration, coagulated blood is applied to both the impaled object and to the laceration. Use gravity to let the blood flow from

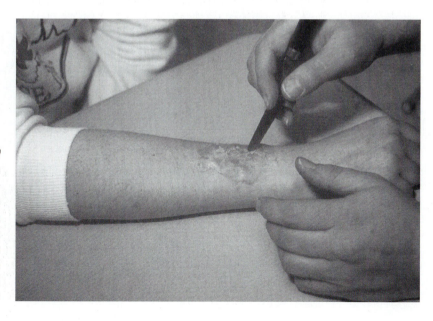

Figure 13-9
Using the artist's knife or a tongue-blade edge, cut the simulated laceration into the wax. Pull the wax out of the cut to add an edge to the cut. (*Photo by Richard Gibbons, Jr.*)

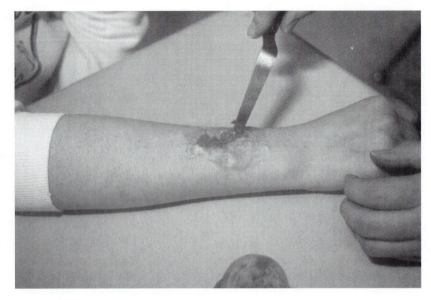

Figure 13-10
Once the laceration has been cut into the wax, red grease liner or red fingernail polish can be applied inside the laceration. (*Photo by Richard Gibbons, Jr.*)

the wound (Figure 13-12). Only apply the blood after the patient actor is fully positioned. Otherwise, the blood flow may not match the simulation.

Moulage Wounds   Stick-on moulage wounds are preformed wounds that are applied directly onto the patient actor's skin (Figure 13-13). A thin coating of glue or double-sided tape will hold the wounds in place. These simulated wounds vary in size, usually from 1 inch to 6 inches in length. When simulation blood is added, the wounds take on a very realistic appearance. These wounds can be used with plasteline or wax.

Fastener-type wounds are less realistic than the stick-on wounds. Fastener-type wounds are positioned onto arms, legs, face, back, and chest. An adjustable strap holds them in place. The patient actor's clothing can be

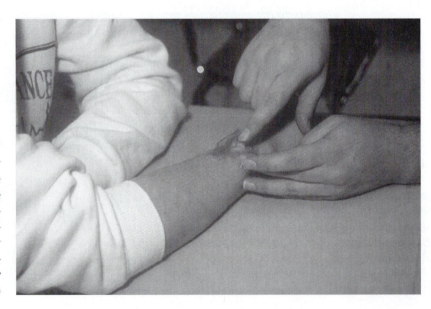

Figure 13-11
Here the instructor has inserted a piece of plexiglass into the laceration. The plexiglass needs to be secured on the sides by the wax from the laceration. (*Photo by Richard Gibbons, Jr.*)

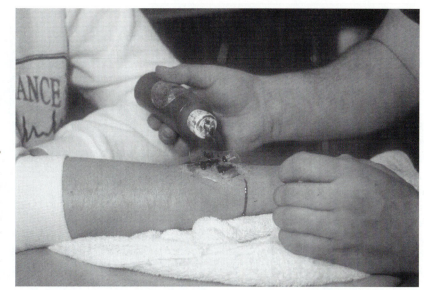

Figure 13-12
Simulated blood is being placed onto the laceration and piece of plexiglass. Let the blood flow naturally out of the laceration. (*Photo by Richard Gibbons, Jr.*)

placed over them and then cut to disclose the wound (Figure 13-14). Many of these devices have bleeder lines that allow blood bags to be connected to the wounds. The patient actor can squeeze a pumping device to simulate an arterial bleeding injury. Because of the bulky nature of these moulage devices, they have lost favor with many instructors. The plastic and fake appearance of these wounds does not render the amount of realism that the other types of makeup and moulage devices provide.

Bleeding   To make a laceration look even more realistic, use a combination of bleeding bags, simulated blood, warmed red latex gel, and coagulated blood. For venous bleeding, use the coagulated blood, thick simulated

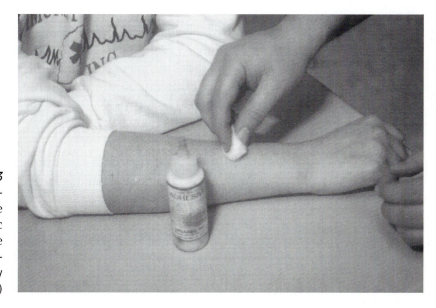

Figure 13-13
Latex adhesive is applied directly to the skin. Then the plastic moulage wounds are applied onto the adhesive. (*Photo by Richard Gibbons, Jr.*)

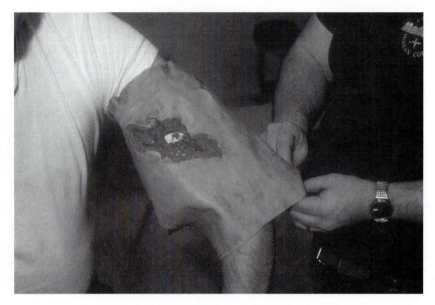

Figure 13-14
Fastener-type
moulage can be
used with bleeding
bags to simulate arte-
rial bleeding. Cloth-
ing can be placed
over the moulage to
hide the moulage.
(*Photo by Richard
Gibbons, Jr.*)

blood, or red latex gel. For arterial bleeding, a bleeding bag with simulated blood is used. Bleeding bag lines can be hidden underneath a wound. The line can be taped onto the patient actor; then the plasteline or wax is applied, and an impaled object or bone fragment is applied on top of the line. The patient actor then simulates severe arterial bleeding when students begin the simulation. The bleeding needs to look realistic and be appropriate for the scenario. Note: Avoid getting simulated blood onto human hair or onto clothing. Simulated blood products do stain.

Abrasions

Abrasions do not require extensive preparation or creativity. Using a stipple sponge and red grease liner can make abrasions. Depending on the scenario, additional black or brown color and dirt or charcoal can be added as a final touch. Even some dabs of simulated blood add realism to the injury.

    Let's look at an example, a motorcycle accident victim. A motorcycle accident victim might have dirt and grass imbedded into the abrasion. To add additional realistic qualities put pieces of dirt or grass into an abrasion. Then rip the patient actor's clothing in the areas of the abrasions. Make the clothing fit the injury. Let creativity flow and create a realistic-looking injury!

Bruises

A variety of bruises can be made from various makeup supplies. Grease liners (blue, red, yellow) can be used individually or mixed together. Eye shadow liners (blue, dark red, green, yellow) can be applied with cosmetic brushes and mixed together (Figure 13-15).

    If a bruise is several days old, it will take on a yellowish-green coloring, combined with a dark blue or purple coloring. Eyeliner colors of yellow, green, and purple can be applied with a cosmetic brush. Grease liners can be combined together to make different shades of colors. For example, a dab of yellow and blue will make a light shade of green. Apply a light

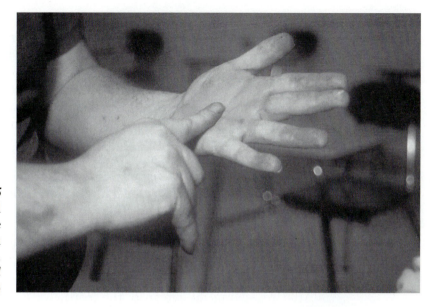

Figure 13-15
Using yellow and
blue grease liners, the
instructor mixes a
week-old bruise.
(*Photo by Richard
Gibbons, Jr.*)

coating of yellow first and then blend it in. Then apply the light green and blend it in. Combining blue and red together makes a light purple color. Apply a small amount of the purple liner to the middle of the bruise site. Both these approaches work equally well to make a realistic bruise.

For more recent bruises, use red and blue colors without any premixing. Blend the colors onto the skin. Apply a red eye shadow or grease liner first, then blend in the blue. Recent bruises have bolder colors than week-old bruises. It becomes very important to determine the type of injury, so the right type of bruise can be made.

Fractures

Both makeup and moulage products provide a variety of possible options. Plasteline, wax, or plastic fastener-type wounds can be used to simulate fractures. Both closed and open fractures can be simulated.

Plasteline or wax can be used to simulate both types of fractures. It is applied and is smoothed out. Then an additional piece is applied on top of the initial coating. Natural coloring is applied to blend it into the patient actor's skin color. A closed fracture should appear swollen and deformed. A compound fracture can have pieces of simulated bone imbedded into the simulated injury. Add several lacerations and simulated blood for the final touch. Even a hidden bleeder line can be added for additional realism.

Moulage fracture wounds, or fastener-type wounds, are alternate devices that can be used to simulate compound fractures. The moulage wounds can be either glued directly to the skin or they can be used with the plasteline or wax. The fastener-style moulage is applied, and clothing is positioned over the moulage. Simulated blood and bleeding bags are used as final touches of realism.

Burns

To do an effective burn simulation, the characteristics of the burn and the setting in which the burn occurred must be known. The scenario directly impacts how a burn is made up. The smell of burned pieces of clothing and hair, combined with the grotesque appearance of the burn itself, makes a burn one of the most emotional injuries for emergency service personnel to treat. These emotional factors can be duplicated through the use of realism concepts.

The scenario must identify the fire setting, time of exposure to the fire source, actions to escape the fire by the victim, and the degree of burns that the victim received. For example, a flash fire victim will probably have burns only to exposed skin surfaces. This would mean portions of the face, ears, neck, legs, and arms. In this type of fire, a person will raise his arms to protect his eyes and face. So the burn area needs to be on the portion of the arm that would have been exposed had the victim raised his arms to cover his face. This is just one example of why it is important for the scenario to guide the instructor through the creation of a burn simulation.

There are numerous ways to simulate a burn (Figure 13-16). The examples that will be discussed are some of the techniques that instructors use. Both makeup and moulaged burns are identified.

After reviewing the scenario, the instructor can identify the type of burns, locations, and other injuries that will be simulated. The first method for creating a burn will be to use makeup products (Figure 13-17). A patient will have varying degrees of burn to an upper right arm as the result of coming in contact with a motorcycle exhaust pipe during an accident. A simulation will need to include a first-, second-, and third-degree burn, dirt and gravel in the burn area and simulated blood coming from the burn area. The burn is the featured injury (Figure 13-18).

For this example, Vaseline, tissue paper, grease liners, charcoal, dirt, and creativity are used. Other makeup items such as liquid latex, clear or scar latex gel, or various moulage devices could be used. The burn area is identified and a thin layer of Vaseline is applied to the area. (Cosmetic mask or other products can be substituted for the Vaseline.) Then ripped pieces of tissue paper are applied to the Vaseline area. An additional thin coat-

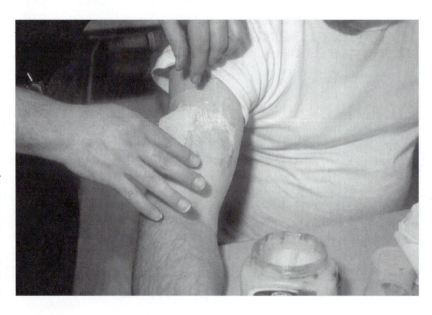

Figure 13-16
Vaseline and tissue paper are the initial components applied for creating a varying degree burn. (*Photo by Richard Gibbons, Jr.*)

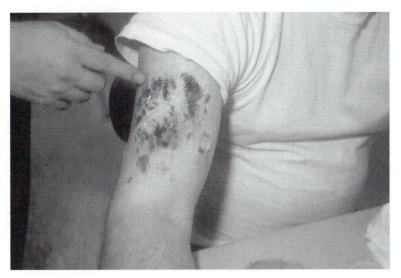

Figure 13-17
Dabs of red, black, and brown grease liners are applied to the burn area. The black and brown colors will be concentrated in the areas of the second- and third-degree burns. (*Photo by Richard Gibbons, Jr.*)

ing of Vaseline is applied on top of the tissue paper. Using a pencil or pen, begin to lift up the tissue paper into little mounds and place small tears in the paper. This creates second-degree and third-degree burn areas. Next add color to the wound. Red grease liner is used to add both the first-degree areas as well as to create localized trauma. Taking dabs of the liner and dotting the outer area of the burn can add the red coloring to the burn. Then, both brown and black grease liners are used to highlight the second- and third-degree burn areas. Dirt and gravel are added to the entire burn area. The finishing makeup is to apply coagulated blood.

This burn is not yet complete. Additional realism, such as burned clothing and hair, contributes the sense of smell to the burn (Figure 13-19). As grotesque as a burn looks, the smell of burned clothing and hair is overpowering to many rescuers. These realism factors are added by burning

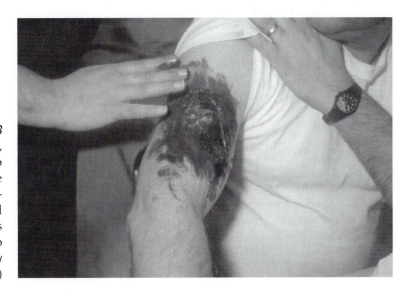

Figure 13-18
As colors are added, the burn begins to take on its grotesque appearance. Simulated blood, dirt, and charcoal are items still to be added to the burn. (*Photo by Richard Gibbons, Jr.*)

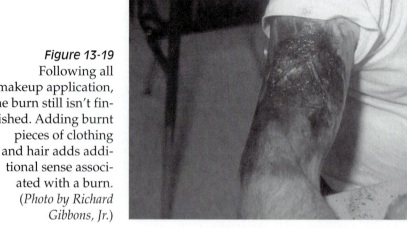

Figure 13-19
Following all
makeup application,
the burn still isn't fin-
ished. Adding burnt
pieces of clothing
and hair adds addi-
tional sense associ-
ated with a burn.
(*Photo by Richard
Gibbons, Jr.*)

portions of clothing that will be used for the scenario. Burned hair clippings can be placed in a dish near the patient actor, or they can be laid on top of the simulated burn. These finishing touches will create a burn simulation that is as close to being real as most rescuers will ever want to encounter.

Creating a burn, as in the previous example, takes a great deal of time. Often instructors may not have the time to make up a burn. Moulage wounds and fastener-type burns may be the answer. Although not as realistic, they can provide some sense of realism.

Amputations

Both makeup and moulage are used to create an amputation. Additionally, various props that simulate amputated body parts are used. Combining these together, realistic-looking injuries are made (Figure 13-20).

Moulage fastener amputations are used to simulate arm and leg amputations. For arm amputations, the patient actor's arm is placed into a flexed position and taped in place. The moulage fastener amputation is placed over the bent elbow and arm. The moulaged arm is placed into the shirt sleeve. The result is only the amputated stump appearing from the shirt sleeve. A bleeding bag can be used to simulate arterial bleeding from the amputation. A fake hand or forearm can be positioned near the patient actor. Simulated blood can be applied to it to add some realism.

Makeup products too can effectively simulate an amputated body part. For example, a thumb amputation can be easily created using some wax, tape, grease liners, simulated blood, and a simulated thumb (Figure 13-21).

The patient actor's thumb is flexed inward toward the palm. Tape is used to hold it in place. A piece of wax is molded onto the bent thumb. Natural grease coloring is blended into the wax to match the patient actor's skin color. Then red liner is added to the bent thumb to simulate the detached portion. Simulated blood is added to finish the realism. The fake thumb is placed near the patient actor. The rest of the realism is up to the patient actor to simulate.

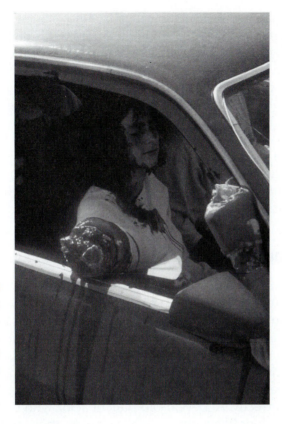

Figure 13-20
A patient-actor is shown with an amputated right arm. Using fastener-type moulage and props, a realistic-looking injury can be created.

Sucking Chest Wound

The sucking chest wound is probably one of the easiest simulations to create. Using plasteline or wax, an Alka-Seltzer tablet, and some simulated blood can create a sucking chest wound. The plasteline or wax is applied to the chest. A depression the size of a nickel is made into the wax. Break pieces of an Alka-Seltzer tablet off and insert them into the depression. Pour several drops of diluted simulated blood onto the tablet and watch the area bubble. One tablet may last up to 45 minutes.

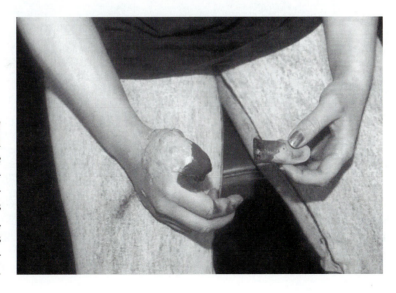

Figure 13-21
An amputated thumb and stump are shown before the application of simuluated blood. It takes good makeup, moulage, and props for an effective amputation scenario.

Associated with a sucking chest wound is often subcutaneous emphysema. There is a nifty way to simulate this condition by using plastic packing air bubbles. Position a sheet of these bubbles onto the chest. Then have the patient actor wear a shirt over the bubbles. As a student assesses the chest region, the bubbles will pop and move around just like real subcutaneous emphysema. This finding will help the students identify the sucking chest wound.

The use of makeup and moulage provides only half the components. The use of appropriate surroundings adds realism (Figure 13-22). But a component that is even more important is the acting ability of the patient actors. Without incorporating all these factors into a simulation, realism will be lost.

Patient Actors and the Surroundings

Aside from makeup and moulage, using patient actors and having good physical surroundings will create realism (Figure 13-23). Not every simulation should be held in a classroom. If students are to experience true realism, realistic patient actors and surroundings are necessary.

Based on a written scenario, a patient actor is selected, programmed, made up, and positioned in an appropriate environment. The patient actor needs to be the right sex and age and, most important, able to portray the scenario correctly. A 15-year-old patient actor who has too much makeup, lays on the floor like a lump, displays no emotion, and is portraying an elderly patient or a scenario that calls for a bathroom setting but is being performed in the middle of the classroom are examples of inappropriate uses of a patient actor and the surroundings. The patient actor's personal display of acting skills should be appropriate for the scenario. If a man has a fractured femur, he is usually in severe pain. He yells out in distress and screams loudly when the leg or body is slightly moved. Patient actors need

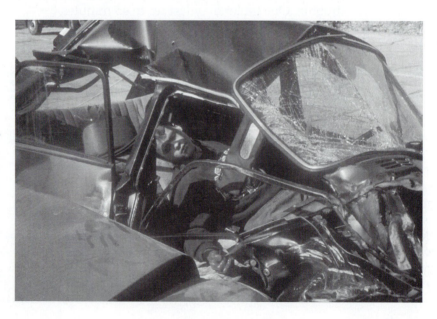

Figure 13-22
The use of makeup and moulage are only half of the components of a simulation. The surroundings and patient-actor's skills are the other components that contribute to realism.

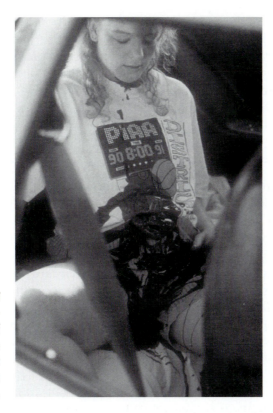

Figure 13-23
A patient's surroundings and the type of patient-actor that is used directly affect the realism of a simulation.

to display this same realism when being treated. Conversely, the patient actor needs to display the correct responses to the student's assessments. Based on the scenario, a patient actor may become unconscious on direction from the instructor. The actors must be briefed in reference to the entire scenario. Any medical history, allergies, medicines, chief complaints, and the onset of the symptoms need to be known by the patient actor. The instructor needs to assess the patient actor's vital signs. This is done to assure that the students are correctly assessing the patient actor's vital signs. These elements make the patient actor believable and realistic.

The patient actor needs to have an additional element, appropriate surroundings. If a patient actor is simulating a drug overdose patient, the setting is enhanced if drug paraphernalia is found lying around the simulation scene. Placing a patient with gastrointestinal bleeding inside a small bathroom setting is more realistic than in the middle of a classroom. Placing props and the patient in an appropriate setting completes the elements needed for effective realism.

Additional Realism Concepts

There are additional realism concepts that can be addressed. The purpose of this chapter was to introduce the concept of realism in educational settings. Drug overdose patients, cardiac emergencies, gunshot wounds, evulsions, abdominal eviscerations, and a host of other conditions can be effectively simulated. The eight or so simulations presented in this chapter can be used to create any of these other conditions. Insert the CD-ROM and click on Realism.

Some training institutes have set up actual pieces of emergency equipment inside the classroom. From having a fully operational modular portion of an ambulance to an operational fire engine pumping panel, some classrooms have taken the need for realism to heart.

Summary

Adult learners require a realistic learning experience. Instructors have a responsibility to include realistic learning experiences in their presentations. Realism not only includes makeup and moulage, it encompasses the surroundings, patient actors, teaching aids, and creativity on the behalf of the instructor.

Multiple cosmetic and moulage products are available. These components are used to create the injuries and symptoms that are identified by the scenario. Without effective acting by the patient actor, the best makeup has only a mild impact. The patient actor needs to act out the scenario. To help the actor, props are used to make the scenario come to life.

The emergency service training facilities themselves are filled with realism. Firefighting students enter burn buildings to rescue trapped victims and extinguish the real fires burning inside the building. High-angle rescue students rappel off training buildings to practice their rappelling skills. EMS students practice extricating injured victims from inside wrecked vehicles. These are all realistic concepts that instructors use and do not even think twice about.

The more realistic a learning experience becomes, the better the overall learning experience becomes. Since adult learners learn best by doing, the ultimate goal becomes to make the learning experience as realistic as possible. It is what learning is all about.

Chapter 14

Legal Aspects of Instruction

➤ OBJECTIVES

- Define the concepts associated with liability:
  - —Identify the forms and elements of negligence.
  - —Identify the degrees of negligence.
  - —Identify the term *standard of care.*
  - —Identify potential liabilities of training personnel.
  - —Discuss sexual harassment in educational settings.
- Explain federal rules and regulations affecting educational institutions:
  - —Define *discrimination.*
  - —Describe the concepts associated with the fair labor standards.
  - —Describe the main points of the Buckley Amendment.
  - —Describe the Americans With Disabilities Act (ADA).
- Identify operational regulations affecting education:
  - —Identify contractual issues affecting educational institutes.
  - —Discuss issues associated with confidentiality.
  - —Identify the importance of documentation.
- Define the importance of adequate individual and institutional liability insurance.

Instructors, even with the best intentions, are potential targets for litigation. Training institutes concern themselves with risk management, sometimes more than they concern themselves with the education of students. So, what programs are safe to teach? This is a question that is being asked by more and more educators (Figure 14-1).

Instructors need to be aware of their potential liabilities. This chapter will provide an overview of potential liabilities facing instructors and training institutes.[1]

Litigation is occurring in instruction. The cost of proving that someone is innocent can be considerable. Many instructors and training institutes do not have any liability insurance. Risk management programming does not exist in many training institutes. Who pays to defend an instructor is not addressed until an incident happens, and then the instructor may end up defending himself.

Note: This chapter is not designed to be an inclusive discussion of instructional liability issues. Law is not simple: It is difficult to be specific concerning the variety of legal interpretations. This chapter is designed to

---

[1]Richard A. Hernan, Jr., Esq. shared his legal expertise and assisted with research and development of this chapter.

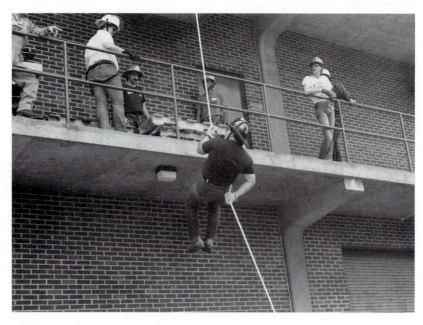

Figure 14-1
How secure are instructors on the liability rope? What are an instructor's risks having this student hanging on this rope? Who pays the medical bills and compensation if this student falls off the rope?

increase an instructor's awareness of potential liabilities. For specific legal issues involving instructors or training institutes, appropriate legal counsel should be sought.

Liability

Liability can be defined as a responsibility that individuals assume, or might assume, when they act, or do not act, in a given situation.[2] An instructor who did not check the training equipment before it was used might be liable if a student is injured as a result of the equipment breaking. So, how does an instructor know if there is any liability? One way is to identify if any negligent acts have occurred. The legal concept of *negligence* applies to many areas of EMS instruction. Let's examine the general concept of negligence.

Negligence is the failure to use reasonable care to avoid foreseeable harm to a person or thing. An individual can be liable if his or her act or failure to act causes injury, even if the harm is unintentional. There are generally four elements that must be present before a court will deem that negligence has occurred:

1. There must be a duty owed. In driving, for example, we owe a duty to others on the road to drive according to the rules of the road. As EMS instructors, we owe our students several duties, examples of which will be discussed later.
2. There must be a breach of the duty. Someone must be able to show that our actions or inactions violated our duty to others. To use the driving example, it must be shown that we have disobeyed the

[2]Reader's Digest, *Legal Question and Answer Book* (Pleasantville, N.Y.: Reader's Digest, 1982) p. 14–213.

rules of the road by driving on the wrong side of the road or failing to stop at a stop signal.
3. The breach of duty must cause the harm to someone.
4. The person must actually be harmed.

What kind of duties do EMS instructors owe the students? Perhaps most obvious is the **duty to provide a safe learning environment.** The classroom and access to the classroom must be safe and well maintained. Stairways must be well lit and free of debris. A training facility must meet or exceed local fire and safety codes.

Vehicle rescue classes pose very difficult problems, both to those practicing the extrication, and to those acting as victims. A student may be injured just as badly in extrication practice as in an actual extrication situation.

Equipment must be sturdy and free of hazards. Training is no place for outdated, overused equipment, such as backboards or ropes. Instructors must be vigilant to not only teach body substance isolation techniques to students but to practice those techniques within the training programs. Infectious diseases can be spread among students using CPR manikins or improper care of needles. The bottom line is for instructors to practice what they preach.

Instructors should not ask students to perform lifts and carries that they might not be able to do without suffering a personal injury. A student should be provided a functional job description for a training course. An instructor should not have training activities exceed a student's aptitudes of performance, based upon the program's functional job description.

An instructor must be vigilant to ensure that sexual assaults do not occur during the close personal contact that occurs in emergency service training programs. Inadvertent contact sometimes occurs. Training programs that allow minors to attend should inform parents of the type of training activities that their children will be participating in. Instructors have a **duty to warn** students or parents of the risks involved in emergency service training programs. EMS, rescue, and fire training is risky business. Instructors must warn students of when they can be hurt. Many students are young or inexperienced. These students have a blind trust in their instructors.

Standard of Care

To assist in proving a negligence case, often the term *standard of care* is identified. This is a measure of comparison that is used to judge an individual's actions, or nonactions, in a situation. These actions are based upon a typical response that a normal individual would have conducted.[3]

The standard of care principle is usually based upon nationally accepted guidelines. For example, EMT training programs use the U.S. Department of Transportation National Standard Curriculum as the basis for teaching the EMT course. Students trained in Florida are held to the same

---

[3]George D. Pozgar, *Legal Aspects of Health Care Administration*, 3rd ed. (Rockville, Md.: Aspen, 1986).

level of training that students in Oregon attain. Although there are differences among the various states, the national curriculum is viewed as the minimum standard of performance. How an EMT performs a particular treatment will be based upon the national standard curriculum and any other state or local protocols that surpass the national curriculum.

From an instructional perspective, an instructor too must meet a "standard of instruction." For example, in the case of a rescue instructor who does not properly show a student how to tie a knot, then allows the student to rappel, and subsequently, the student falls from the rope, there is a good chance that there is negligence on the instructor's part. Instructors must teach lesson material according to the lesson plans and to the curriculum used by a training institute.

Sexual Harassment

Emergency service classes bring together a wide variety of students and teachers in classroom situations that encourage physical contact. The stage is set for claims of sexual harassment.

Sexual harassment takes many forms, and the behaviors defined as harassing are ever expanding. Sexual harassment victims may be either students or teachers. What, then, is sexual harassment?

A clear type of sexual harassment occurs when a teacher either expressly or by implication makes an educational decision concerning the student dependent on the student's submission to unwelcome sexual advances, requests for sexual favors, or other conduct of a sexual nature. This is known as quid pro quo harassment. Sexual harassment can also occur when verbal or physical conduct of a sexual nature is so pervasive, severe, and persistent that it creates a hostile environment. Conduct that has been deemed sexually harassing includes: jokes or pictures of a sexual nature, remarks about a person's body or sexual activities, repeated brushing up against a person's body, subtle or open pressure for sexual favors, and other sexually oriented behavior. Sexual harassment of the first type, quid pro quo, generally takes place where the teacher is the harasser and the student is the victim. Sexual harassment of the second type, hostile environment sexual harassment, however, can occur between teachers and students, students and teachers, students and students, and of course, teachers and teachers.

Emergency classes are generally adult education classes open to a wide range of students from those who are minors to those who are retired. Additionally, emergency service organizations recruit volunteers, many of them minors, to act as patients for examinations and drills. Many times, the backgrounds of those participating in the classes are unknown. There is, therefore, a wide range of sexual sophistication and experience in a typical class (Figure 14-2).

As already noted, emergency classes encourage close physical contact among those involved. Nearly every aspect of emergency training, including hands-on assessment and treatment of a patient, performing drags and carries, and SCBA buddy-breathing training, requires physical contact. In

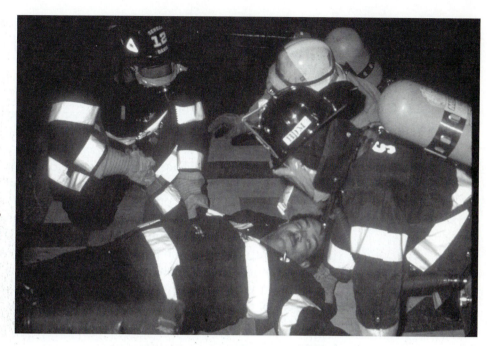

Figure 14-2
Not every injury that is sustained in a class is an act of negligence. Instructors need to minimize the risk of injury wherever possible.

another situation these behaviors would otherwise be considered offensive and prohibited. The law will recognize and permit such physical contact under certain circumstances without it being deemed sexual harassment. The students should be forewarned, however, about the physical contact that will happen and the fact that contact with personal body parts may occur. Parents of minors should likewise be warned about this potential. Every effort should be made to ensure that the students and teachers treat each other with courtesy and respect.

Prevention, of course, is the key to avoiding problems of allegations of sexual harassment. Each training institute should have a comprehensive and well-communicated policy against sexual harassment. That policy should sensitize all involved to the problem, express strong disapproval of sexual harassment, and have meaningful sanctions. There should be a procedure for resolving sexual harassment complaints. The procedure should be confidential and should not require that the offending behavior be reported first to the offending supervisor or teacher. Mandatory education and training of all instructors should be done and all students should be given a copy of the policy and the procedure for raising complaints at the beginning of each course.

One further area of risk occurs when a student is outside of the instructor's presence doing clinical or field training. Whether the clinical or field experience takes place in a hospital, ambulance service, or any other location, the potential exists for the student to be sexually harassed. The students must be made aware that they are covered by the institute's training policy no matter where the training is taking place.

Sexual harassment issues are and will continue to be a serious risk for emergency service educators, given the nature of the instruction. Just as in other areas, such as communicable diseases, emergency vehicle operations, and medication errors, the risks are reduced with well-informed and well-communicated policies.

Laws and Regulations

Laws and regulations apply to nearly every human activity in our country, and emergency service education is no exception. Laws as familiar as the Wage-and-Hour provisions of the Fair Labor Standards Act to those as unfamiliar as the Family Educational Rights and Privacy regulations under the General Education Provisions Act may have a bearing on an emergency service training institute's policies and programs. What follows is just a brief overview of some of the more important laws and regulations. Many of the federal laws set out below apply only when there are a minimum number of employees. Much more information is available on the Internet, in libraries, and through each state's emergency service offices. There is, of course, no substitute for a consultation with an attorney knowledgeable in these areas of the law.

DISCRIMINATION

Federal laws prohibiting discrimination in employment have been on the books for nearly 40 years. State laws, which may be even more restrictive, are also in effect. An employer may not discriminate on the basis of race, color, religion, sex, or national origin.[4] There can be no wage discrimination between men and women in substantially the same job in the same workplace.[5] There can be no discrimination against persons 40 years of age or older.[6] Discrimination on the basis of citizenship is prohibited.[7] The relatively new but critically important Americans with Disabilities Act protects an otherwise qualified individual with a disability from discrimination, and sets out the responsibilities of employers to accommodate disabled persons.[8] Training institutes should adopt functional job descriptions for training programs that comply with the ADA and other federal and state statutes.

FAIR LABOR STANDARDS

EMS training institutes must be familiar with the Fair Labor Standards Act which sets out the minimum wage and overtime standards, as well as the child labor rules for employers.[9] So too, employers must be aware of the

---

[4]Civil Rights Act of 1964, Title VII, Public Law 88-352, Volume 42, United States Code. Amended 1991, Public Law 102-166.

[5]Equal Pay Act of 1963, Public Law 88-38, Volume 2 of United States Code, Section 206.

[6]Age Discrimination in Employment Act of 1977, Public Law 90-202, Volume 29, United States Code Section 621.

[7]Immigration Reform and Control Act, 1986, IRCA, Public Law 99-603.

[8]Americans With Disabilities Act 1990, Public Law 101-336, Statue 327, Section 42, United States Code 12101.

[9]Fair Labor Standards Act 1938, Section 201-219, Title 29, United States Code.

Family Medical Leave Act which requires employers to provide a limited amount of leave to employees with serious illness of themselves or a family member and the birth or adoption of a child.[10]

BUCKLEY AMENDMENT

Instructors should be aware of an important federal law called the Family Educational Rights and Privacy Act (20 U.S.C. § 1232g; 34 CFR Part 99), which is known as FERPA and also called the Buckley Amendment. This law was passed by Congress in 1974 and contains important rules for educational institutes that receive federal funds through the U.S. Department of Education.

This law grants students over the age of 18 the following rights:

- A student, or if the student is under 18, the parent, has the right to inspect and review the student's educational records that are maintained by the school.
- A student, or if the student is under 18, the parent, has the right to request that the school correct records that they think are inaccurate or misleading. If the school refuses to amend the record, the student or parent has the right to request a formal hearing. If, after the hearing, the school still refuses to amend the record, the student or parent has the right to place a statement in the student's record with the student's or parent's version of the contested information.
- Importantly, students have a right to confidentiality of their educational records. If the student is over 18, not even the parents have a right to this information without the student's permission.

There are, of course, exceptions to the confidentiality rule, which may permit the release of the student's educational information. A quick review of the law at the Department of Education (DOE) website will allow the instructor to see if an exception applies to any particular request.

An educational institution may disclose "directory information" without the students' consent. This information is limited to names, addresses, dates of birth, honors, and so forth and does not include any information about the courses taken and grades received. A student may refuse permission to the institution regarding the release of even this directory information.

Institutes must advise all students of their rights under FERPA at least annually. This may be done through letters, student handbooks, or other materials, but it is important to ensure that every student gets the information.

Public discussion of students' scores is prohibited. Discussion of students' results with third-party instructors is not permitted. Posting or orally

---

[10]Family Medical Leave Act 1993, Public Law 103-3, Title 29, United States Code 2601.

reading students' scores by an individual's name is not permitted. Suspending a student without reasonable due process is a violation. The list of examples can go on and on. This law was implemented in 1974, and yet in many training institutes, some of these practices still exist. If an instructor or training institute is openly abusing these statutes, they may have a serious liability issue.

Operational Regulations

The following are laws or regulations that influence educational systems either directly or indirectly.

CONTRACT THEORY

All students entering an EMS course have the reasonable expectation that the course will prepare them to successfully pass the final exam and to get the certificate or license that they are seeking. Many students leave jobs and enroll in training with hopes of bettering themselves financially or to pursue their favored career. They make many sacrifices to take the courses and often pay substantial amounts of tuition. As consumers, they feel that they are entitled to get what they pay for. If they do not, they may sue.

Under an old doctrine known as academic abstention, courts have been reluctant to get involved in suits brought by students against schools for breach of contract. That reluctance is fading. Courts are recently tending to view education as an industry and applying general principals of contract law to the institution-student relationship. That relationship depends on the reasonable expectations of the parties.

An institution that guarantees or even implies that certain materials will be covered or that certain certifications will be attained at or by the end of the program may be successfully sued. Those guarantees or implications may be found in the course announcements, brochures, catalogs, bulletins, course outlines, student handbooks, or oral expressions of course administrators and teachers. A court may hold that these items and others define the reasonable expectations of the students. The expectations are to be viewed through the eyes of a reasonable student, not the institution.

Standards for the student to continue in a course and to pass the course must be clearly defined. Students must know what is expected of them and how they are doing as a course proceeds. If their performance is deficient, they should be given written notice of the deficiencies and of how they can remediate the deficiency. If a student's performance on practical skills is substandard, an independent review by a second or third instructor should be performed. This may help to avoid any claims of personality conflicts.

If students can point to specific deficiencies in the program and show that it falls short of what the institution led them to reasonably expect, they may be successful in a suit against the institution for breach of their contractual agreement.

DOCUMENTATION

An instructor's lesson plan and other types of course paperwork are critical forms of documentation because they specify what an instructor planned to teach. Skill check-off sheets and critique forms help provide instructors with a validation of the abilities of their students. And a written record of a student's performance on written examinations throughout a course is a critical form of documentation.

In addition to these forms of documentation, instructors may want to keep a logbook of their training activities. During the lesson presentation, instructors may overlook certain points from the written lesson plan. They may not even recognize them until they review their presentation notes. Most instructors will jot down these missed points and present them at the next class. After they review the material they throw away the jotted notes. This is where a logbook can save an instructor. Instead of throwing these notes away, save them. A logbook is a great tool for self-evaluation of an instructor's performance and can be an instructor's life preserver when questions are raised regarding course content.

Each time a lesson plan is used, instructors should review how well they followed it. If material was missed, or should have been covered in a different manner, the next time the lesson plan is presented, the instructor will remember to cover those areas. A running list of dates should be included in the lesson plan. Each time the lesson plan is presented or modified, the date should be added to the running list.

Why is all this documentation necessary? First and foremost it should be done as part of an instructor's or training institute's desire for improved instructional performance. But secondly, it should be done as part of a risk-management strategy to provide documentation regarding how a lesson was presented. If students claim they and other students in the class did not receive adequate instruction, these forms of documentation will become critical legal documents for an instructor.

CONFIDENTIALITY

Students in medical programs often participate in clinical or field training. Contact with actual patients is a part of a student's training. During their contact with a patient in either a hospital or field setting, students will be exposed to confidential patient information, and these students, unless formally instructed, could disclose confidential information to other students or friends and breech a patient's confidentiality. This places the instructor, preceptors, training institute, and the clinical/field setting into litigation jeopardy.

Students must be formally instructed on the need to keep patient information confidential. Many students and even instructors do not understand how sensitive patient information can be. They do not understand how much exposure the instructional agencies assume if there is a breech in confidentiality. Unless they are made aware of the importance of protecting a patient's right to privacy, students may breech the confidence and not even know they did. It is up to the instructor of any training program to inform the students to protect the confidentiality of patient information.

Instructional Insurance

This is not a commercial for liability insurance; rather, it is designed to be a life-saving plan for an instructor. All instructors should be aware that they have a risk of someone being injured in the training program. Even though it may not be an instructor's fault, the case of proving it was not the instructor's fault can be an expensive venture. Court costs, lawyers' fees, loss of pay due to court appearances, and the potential damages that may be awarded from a court case are significant. Many training institutes may not have any, or minimal, liability coverage. The instructor may not even be covered by the institute's policy. An instructor may very well be risking his family's house, car, and lifestyle as a result of a court awarded settlement. Instructors and training institutes need to limit their risks. Implementing a risk management program within a training institute is one way to reduce liability exposure. Some forms of liability cannot be avoided. Adequate insurance coverage for both an instructor and the training institute becomes a necessity.

Instructors love teaching (Figure 14-3). They teach on nights and weekends they have off because they want to share their knowledge and experi-

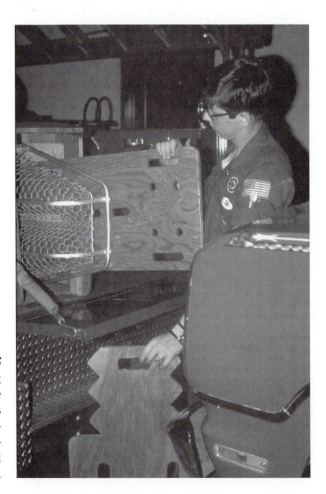

Figure 14-3
Inspecting training equipment before live practice sessions helps to assure student safety and reduces potential liability exposure.

ences with others. This idealistic perception is shattered when someone gets injured. Instructors who have not planned for a court case may find themselves missing their full-time employment to meet with lawyers and attend court sessions. Thousands of dollars in attorney fees and court costs can be accumulated—just to prove that an instructor was innocent.

Fortunately, liability insurance plans have been designed for instructors. They have a wide range of premiums, usually according to the degree of liability that an instructor will have when instructing. An avid instructor should consider to include, as an expense of teaching, personal liability insurance.

Instructors should ask their training institute about how much liability coverage is provided to instructors. Specifically, they should ask how much coverage they will receive from the policy. Many policies do not pay lawyer fees and court costs that an instructor may incur in defending a lawsuit. The plan may cover only the institute, leaving the instructor totally uncovered.

It is unfortunate that instructors face these liabilities. However, this is a part of instruction that will not improve until other societal values change. Instructors should look out for themselves before a lawsuit is filed. Insurance is viewed as an instructor's form of risk management. Liability insurance becomes an instructor's safety net.

Summary

Instructing is not as easy as just writing a lesson plan and standing in front of a group of students. There are multiple issues that instructors must be aware of before they even begin to write a lesson plan. Knowing the legal issues associated with a particular form of emergency training is one of these issues.

Instructors and training institutes are liable for various aspects of the training programs. Federal, state, and civil laws dictate how instructors can teach students.

Instructors are often employees of a training institute. The training institute must follow employment related regulations that are mandated by the federal and state governments. National agencies provide standards of instruction that are used to train personnel.

Instructors are potential targets for litigation. Instructors and training institutes can form risk management groups to try to limit potential liabilities. But the instructor often is left uncovered in the legal sense. If charged with an offense, many training institute liability policies do not provide a blanket coverage to individual instructors. Instructors could be faced with thousands of dollars of legal fees, just to prove their innocence. Personal liability insurance should be considered by instructors as a safety net for their personal livelihood.

Emergency service training programs need competent and experienced instructors (Figure 14-4). A reaction after reading this chapter might be to throw in the towel: "The risks are not worth the benefits." The intention of this chapter is not to drive instructors out of the business. Rather, it

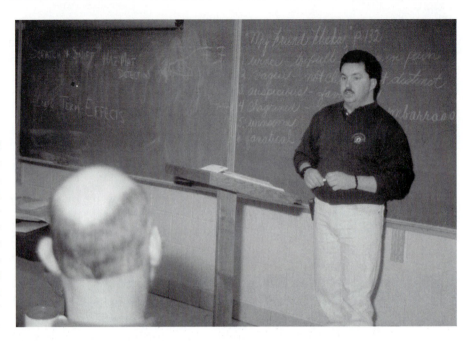

Figure 14-4
Emergency service training programs need competent and experienced instructors. In today's litigious society, the altruistic desires of instructors must be balanced with personal liability concerns.

is to make instructors aware of potential liabilities. While there are documented cases of negligence that have been filed against training institutes and instructors, these cases are rarely found in trade journals. Instructors who teach to the national standards, document their instruction, and provide a safe learning environment are not high-risk targets. It is when an instructor does not teach the correct information or provides an unsafe learning environment that potential liabilities increase.

The bottom line is that there are legal risks in teaching emergency service training programs. Instructors need to accept this fact and minimize the liabilities that they can. It is a part of teaching that instructors must be aware of. It is an issue that most instructors who conduct training programs should never have to face, but if they do, it is hoped they have a safety net in place to protect their livelihood.

Chapter 15

Program Administration

➤ OBJECTIVES

- Identify administrative procedures associated with operating a program.
- Explain the approaches used in handling disruptive students in a training program.
- Stress the need for due process when using disciplinary measures.
- Identify the roles associated with a course coordinator.
- Identify the roles and responsibilities of a training administrator.
- Describe the interface between the instructors and the administrators.
- Discuss the paperwork that may be required by many courses.
- Describe the process used to develop a budget for a course.
- Explain funding, other than student tuition, for operating a training program.
- Explain how training institutes advertise and promote a program.
- Assure program quality throughout a training program.
- Explain the extra perks for students in a course.
- Discuss the need for training institute personnel to keep abreast of laws, curriculum updates, and state/federal regulations that affect the training institute.
- Discuss the accreditation of training institutes.

Exactly how is a training program set up? Who decides to run a program? How many people are allowed to enroll? What is the minimal passing score on written examinations? Who advertises the program? What curriculum is used? These types of questions go on and on. However, the answer to most of these questions is the same: Program administration.

Behind every program, there is a network of individuals who are responsible for its success or failure. These people are covered under an umbrella called program administration. Who are these people? What do they do? What impact do they have on a training program? These are the main questions addressed in this chapter.

Program Administrative Procedures

For an instructor to present a quality program takes more than just a dynamic personality and presentation (Figure 15-1). To conduct an entire course takes a lot of planning and administrative effort. Actually, more planning and preparation goes into the administrative phase than goes

265

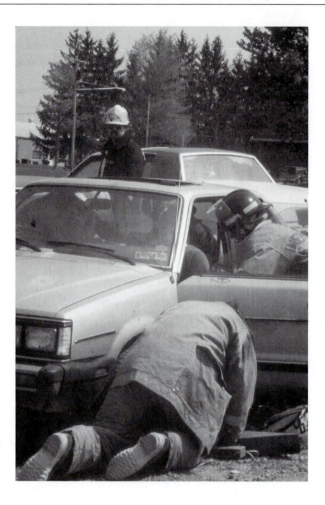

Figure 15-1
A lot of planning and preparation goes into conducting a rescue course besides writing lesson plans.

into preparing a lesson presentation. Whether it is an EMS, fire, or rescue program, a variety of program details fall under the program administration umbrella.

A policy manual is an effective adjunct to oversee the administrative aspects of a training institute. Included in a policy manual are:

- Program mission statement
- Administrative titles
- Course title/descriptions
- Listing of instructors
- Disciplinary procedures
- Records and reporting (forms)
- Flow chart of responsibility
- Job descriptions
- Teaching curriculum
- Inventory of equipment
- Accreditation materials
- Quality improvement initiatives
- Financial/budget

These are some of the items that may be found in a typical manual. There are additional items that can be included in a manual of this type. It is important that both the administration and instructors participate in the development of a policy manual. Policy and procedures that are jointly developed stand a better chance of being followed than those that reflect only one side's opinions.

A well-written manual provides the instructors, course coordinator, and training administration with the same set of policies to follow. When a question arises, the first place that is referenced is the policy manual. For most situations, the policy manual should answer most questions. If it does not, the administration should be asked for an opinion or interpretation.

A policy manual sets standards for a training institute. To understand how a manual is developed, the following section looks at the list of policy manual components and identifies the key elements from the previous list.

Mission Statement

The mission statement is usually located in the first several pages of a manual. This is a brief set of sentences that state the purpose and chief goals that the training institute has identified for its personnel and students to accomplish. A well-written mission statement should be no more than a few paragraphs in length.

The mission statement is often used as the focal point for both short- and long-term goals. What the training institute is accomplishing today may be the beginning of a long-range goal for tomorrow. The mission statement outlines these immediate and far-reaching goals for the institute.

An essential element of the mission statement deals with quality. For example, what are the minimal performance standards being established by the institute? The mission statement needs to answer this question and leave no doubts to the minimum performance standards that will be accepted.

Institute Administration

Three major categories fall into this broad category called institute administration. These are administration titles, specific job descriptions, and a visual listing of job responsibilities. The following titles, job descriptions, and responsibility chart are intended to be generic. Often, many of the job descriptions and responsibilities will be shared by several individuals. It is important that instructors identify the administrative structure for their specific training institute. Use the following information as a guide to identify who does what within a training institute.

Who are the players under the title of administration? The following are some of the commonly found titles, or jobs, associated with a training institute:

- Executive director/dean
- Clerical
- Training administrator
- Instructors (primary and secondary)

- Equipment maintenance (for training equipment)
- Specialty personnel (guest lecturers, preceptors, medical directors, etc.)
- Financial department
- Facility maintenance
- Course coordinators

Figure 15-2 shows a flow of responsibility for a typical training institute.

Each of these positions can influence how a training program is conducted. For example, if an instructor needs handout material copied and the clerical staff is not able to copy the materials the instructor will not be able to present the lesson material as planned. Any one of the positions can influence the performance of the entire training institute.

"Who does what tasks" is important to know. The following are brief job descriptions for each of the categories identified in Figure 15-2.

EXECUTIVE DIRECTOR/DEAN

Many training institutes are academically linked to a university, community college, or vocational-technical school. In this type of setting, a dean or administrative director will be the individual in charge of the entire emer-

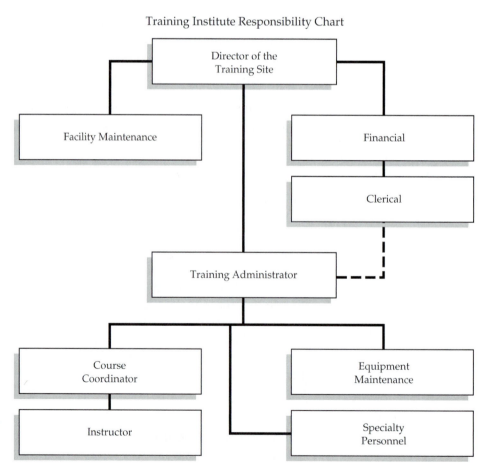

Training Institute Responsibility Chart

Figure 15-2
Training institute responsibility chart.

gency service training institute. Often, an emergency service training institute will be one of several training institutes that are coordinated by this individual.

The physical facilities, facility maintenance, security, accounting/finances, and clerical staff are directly supervised by this individual. The training administrator is supervised by the director. The director must rely on the training administrator to oversee the other personnel in the training institute. Even though delegation of authority is common, the director is still ultimately responsible for any of the personnel's actions.

The director needs to establish and follow administrative policies and procedures that coincide with the mission statement for the training institute. This occurs only when there are open lines of communication among the institute faculty. The director becomes a focal point for the entire institute. When a problem arises that relates to institute policy, the director must render the final decision. Someone is always in charge of an organization, and in a typical training institute this person is the director.

FINANCIAL/ACCOUNTING/PAYROLL

The size of a training institute often determines how these jobs are assigned and accomplished. Training institutes have bills and financial obligations, as does any other business. The financial position is supervised by the executive director. These personnel work closely with the director to assure that funding is sufficient to cover the training program expenditures. In smaller training institutes, the financial personnel often issue payroll and payments for expenses.

In large university settings, the financial department may be an entirely separate entity. In this case, specific training-institute records may be kept and reported to the main financial department for final distribution.

A significant benefit to being part of an established educational institution is the use of in-kind services. Instead of the training institute paying for capital improvements to training facilities, providing building maintenance and security, purchasing business equipment, paying for copying costs, buying audiovisual equipment, and even paying some personnel costs, all can be shared costs among the entire educational institution. When a training institute must pay for each of these individual costs, the result is less funding for improving individual training programs and an increased tuition fee for students.

Accounting for each tuition dollar is essential. The financial personnel help the director coordinate the yearly schedules for the training institute. Only so many programs can be financially operated in a year. From the yearly financial planning to payroll and even to an itemized accounting system for the institute, all are essential for the training institute to exist.

CLERICAL

Much of the training institute operations are dependent upon an efficient clerical staff. Clerical staffs prepare assorted training materials, handle registration materials, process the registration materials, assist tracking students through a training program, record and file course documents, and many more daily tasks that keep the institute functioning.

In smaller institutes, the clerical staff may also assume some of the financial responsibilities. They become responsible for keeping track of daily expenses and keeping the overall financial records and accounting.

FACILITY MAINTENANCE

Directly under the supervision of the director are the personnel needed to keep a facility looking clean (Figure 15-3). Much of a training institute's image relates to the building's maintenance: a dirty floor in a training room can make a negative statement to the students. Well-maintained rooms instill a sense of quality in students and instructors. Assuring the rooms are maintained is another noneducational factor that can affect a training program's quality.

TRAINING ADMINISTRATOR

The day-to-day logistical operations of a training institute are handled by the training administrator. Whether it is coordinating the movement of training equipment from one classroom to another or preparing a six-month training schedule, the training administrator is involved. Some of the tasks a training administrator is involved with are the following:

- Develop the training program schedules
- Establish a budget for each training program; within the budget, establish instructor reimbursement schedules, student tuition fees, and identify any costs involved in the operation of the program
- Identify and secure additional funding for the training programs

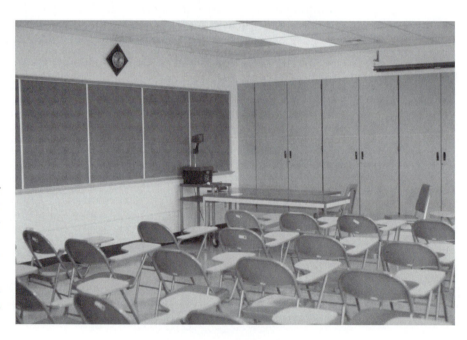

Figure 15-3
Well-maintained classrooms don't happen by accident. Facility maintenance personnel are an asset to training in maintaining room cleanliness.

- Advertise the training programs in the local community
- Hire and supervise the course coordinators, instructors, equipment maintenance personnel, and any other specialty personnel needed for the operation of a training program
- Identify and purchase training equipment for the institute
- Jointly develop training policies with the instructional staff
- Assure that the training programs are complying with the minimum standards of performance for the training institute
- Working with individual course coordinators, assure that instructors have the necessary resources for a training program
- Review course registration materials and instructor reimbursement forms for each training program
- Develop short- and long-term goals for the training institute
- Assume responsibility for any additional tasks as assigned by a director

The training administrator is the logistical engineer for a training program. Any matters dealing with day-to-day operations of the institute find their way to the training administrator's office. Unlike a course coordinator who deals with a single training program, a training administrator may be dealing with multiple training programs. A training administrator learns to balance equipment, personnel, and financial resources to keep a training institute operating efficiently. Without a good logistical administrator, problems tend to occur.

COURSE COORDINATOR

Working with the training administrator, a course coordinator carries out many of the logistics for the training administrator. The course coordinator is the immediate logistics person for a training program. It is the course coordinator who assures the availability of AV equipment, copying handouts, room assignments, field-trip arrangements, or preparing examination booklets for the instructors. Much of a program's training records are kept by the course coordinator. Records like attendance, examination performance, instructor assignments/schedules, clinical/preceptor rotation assignments, and any disciplinary reports are kept by the course coordinator.

If an instructor needs a special facility, like a burn building, the course coordinator assures that the facility is ready for a training program. Training equipment for a program is obtained by the course coordinator. The course coordinator works with the instructors to assure a continuity of instruction. It is the course coordinator who monitors instructor presentations. This is done to assure that the lesson material is being taught to the training institute's standards and that the instructor is using accepted educational techniques. This is a vital quality assurance mechanism used by training institutes.

Both the course coordinator and training administrator positions are vital to the success of a training program. Instructors rely heavily upon these individuals to provide them with instructional resources for their presentations. Without efficient logistical coordination, both the instructors and students end up being affected by their actions. Good logistical coordination by the course coordinator is essential if a quality learning experience is to occur.

INSTRUCTORS

Instructors are the front-line people whom students see on a regular basis (Figure 15-4). They require a significant number of resources to present a training program that works efficiently. The instructor follows the policies that the training institute has established to present the lesson material. Copies of any handout materials, AV supplies, or other education materials are usually available through either the course coordinator or training administrator. The instructor's role is to instruct. Rarely do instructors become involved in the administrative details. Not being involved in administrative activities allows the instructor to concentrate on one mission, instructing.

Because instructors are developing their own materials, many training institutes request a copy of the instructor's lesson plans. The course coordinator reviews them to assure that they are complying with the institute's instructional goals.

The instructors, course coordinators, and the training administrator need to meet together on a regular basis. The institute's educational policies and goals need to be developed and evaluated on a frequent basis. An improved educational experience is possible only if all the instructional staff works together. Seeking input and jointly developing the institute's

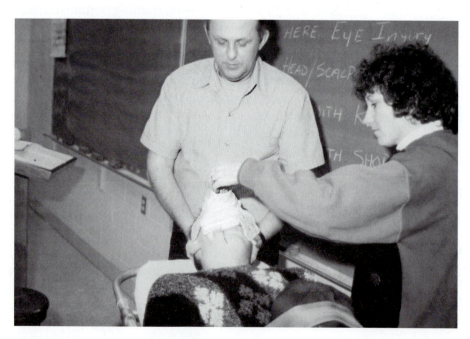

Figure 15-4
Instructors are the front-line personnel of a training institute. What they say and do influences the training institute.

goals are essential for keeping open communications among the instructional staff.

EQUIPMENT MAINTENANCE

Training equipment is heavily used in training programs. When students make mistakes, the equipment often receives the effects of these mistakes. To preserve the life span of the equipment and to assure its safety, training institutes hire equipment maintenance personnel. Whether the equipment is CPR training manikins or ½-inch kernmantle rope, an equipment maintenance person needs to inspect the equipment after each use. In smaller training institutes, the course coordinator or primary instructor acts as the equipment maintenance person.

Potential liability exists for a training institute if the equipment is not properly maintained. Aside from the liability issues, training equipment is expensive. Most training sites cannot afford to buy new equipment every year. The training equipment must be durable and needs to be adequately maintained if yearly replacement purchases are to be avoided.

SPECIALTY PERSONNEL

Based on the type of training programs that a training institute operates, additional staff members may be required. For example, in EMS training institutes, a program medical director, clinical preceptors, and field preceptors are additional personnel who may be required. These preceptors assure that the students complete the required clinical and field components for a training program. The medical director oversees the operation of a training program and assures that the program is providing the proper medical information to the students.

Other specialty personnel may include guest lecturers, usually personnel who specialize in a trade. Police officers, hazardous material personnel, public utility personnel, and stress management personnel are some of the possible specialty personnel included in an emergency service training program. The use of these specialty personnel is coordinated by either the training administrator or the course coordinator. Specific reimbursement fees and any additional logistics are handled without involving the instructor with these tasks.

As you can see, the umbrella of the training administration is quite large. A lot of tasks need to be accomplished before the first training session. There is a lot more to emergency-service training programs than just developing lesson plans and course materials. Instructors need to recognize the personnel with whom they will be interfacing during a training program. Knowing what personnel will help them with specific tasks reduces an instructors' anxiety levels and improves their ability to conduct a quality training program.

Discipline and Performance Standards

Although normally thought of as being for disruptive students, in emergency service training programs the scope of discipline is rather broad. Additionally, a training institute or other governing agency establishes minimum performance standards. For example, if a student does not attain a 70 percent or higher on a midterm examination, the student is to be dropped from a course. Due to the legality of these issues, both discipline and performance standards usually take up a few pages in a policy manual.

Before discussing either of these topics in depth, another concept needs to be discussed. That concept is *due process,* the legal structure that assures the rights of an individual.[1] Within a training institute manual, a specific outline for handling a disciplinary or performance issue must be identified. This outline identifies the actions that an instructor, course coordinator, or training administrator should take for specific problems. A student is not to be terminated from a training program unless there is sufficient documentation that will support a dismissal. Students have the right to appeal. This is where the true meaning of due process occurs. A student must be informed of the appeal process. The student must be given an opportunity to challenge any decision.

Informing the students of their rights becomes a significant aspect of the due process concept. Students need to know the appeal process that is in place for a training institute. Should a disciplinary event occur, the student must be provided both oral and written notice of the problem and allowed to enter the appeal process. Not allowing students the right to challenge a disciplinary action may infringe upon their individual rights and open the potential for legal actions against an institute.

Great care needs to be taken in writing disciplinary and performance standards. Depending upon the type of issue, an immediate dismissal from a training program may be appropriate. Other offenses against students are handled with one-to-one counseling sessions. The following is a list of some of the disciplinary areas and performance standards that many training institutes have identified:

- Sexual harassment
- Psychological abuse
- Theft of property
- Cheating on exams
- Falsification of records
- Failure to maintain a minimum level of performance
- Disruptive actions during a training program
- Physical abuse of other students
- Criminal acts of violence
- Intentional misuse of equipment
- Attendance at training sessions
- Plus many more

---

[1] Reader's Digest, *Legal Question and Answer Book* (Pleasantville, N.Y.: Reader's Digest, 1982).

Some of these offenses are quite serious. More than just a face-to-face meeting is often required. Immediate dismissal or suspension from a training program may be appropriate in some cases. The training institute must decide which offenses warrant immediate action and which do not. Instructors need to know what they are permitted to do when they observe one of these offenses occurring. The policies must be detailed. The actions that are appropriate for an instructor or course coordinator must be identified.

It should be noted that the institute manual should have disciplinary policies not only for students but also for the instructional and administrative staff. It is not unheard of for students to lodge sexual harassment allegations against an instructor or administrator. The person to whom the students should speak about a disciplinary issue involving either an instructor or an administrative staff member needs to be identified. Often students' fears of actions being taken against them stop them from telling anyone about an incident. Students need to be told whom to contact at a training institute when an incident involving the institutional staff occurs. Most important, students need to know that no punitive actions will be taken against them for notifying the institute of a problem.

Most of this discussion has been about the significant disciplinary problems in a training program. But what about the classroom problems that are an annoyance to instructors? Students' excessive talking during class, being late for class sessions, standing around and not practicing, constantly interrupting the instructor during a presentation, smoking during classroom activities, and being know-it-alls are common disciplinary problems that instructors deal with. Handling many of these problems must be done immediately by the instructor.

For example, students who are talking during an instructor's presentation are a disruption for the entire class. An instructor should acknowledge the students who are talking and determine if there is a problem with the material being presented. The instructor should encourage their attention to the presentation and move on in the presentation. If the talking continues, a bolder move is to put the students on the spot by asking them to explain what is being discussed. If these casual techniques do not work, then an instructor should sit down with the students and counsel them on their behavior. An instructor should tell the students that they are interrupting the class and that their conversations are not appropriate during a classroom presentation. A written report of the session should be filed with the course coordinator or training administrator. If the disruptions continue, additional counseling sessions or other disciplinary actions may need to be taken by the institute.

This example shows a typical response used by instructors. This type of response can be used with almost any classroom disruption. Only those disruptions that are of a serious or repetitive nature may enter into the formal disciplinary process.

Written documentation is vital in any disciplinary action. For every training institute, various forms of documentation are used. The next section looks at the types of common forms of written documentation that are associated with training programs.

Written Documentation

A necessary evil of any business is paperwork. Most training programs generate significant training records. Even with a computer filing system, written training records are still kept. The following list identifies some of the commonly found forms of written documentation for a training program:

- Examination results
- Grievance/disciplinary
- Course roster
- Instructor schedules/rosters/reimbursement forms
- Lesson plans
- Clinical training forms
- Skill verification forms
- Attendance records
- Registration forms
- Class registration material
- Tuition payment forms
- Miscellaneous cost forms
- And more . . . and more . . . forms

Both instructors and administrative staff share the responsibilities for assuring the written documentation is completed. Instructors often are requested to complete various forms during a training program. Instructor reimbursement forms, time sheets, student counseling forms, practical examination performance sheets, and written-examination results are types of documentation completed by instructors.

Instructors should be aware of any written documentation that is required for a training program. Aside from development of instructional material, timely completion of administrative paperwork is necessary in most training institutes. Instructors should find out when specific forms need to be submitted. Often an instructor's reimbursement is held up if the paperwork is not submitted on time. Unfortunately, completion of paperwork is a part of being an instructor, and instructors need to get to know the paperwork game for their training institute.

Because some of the paperwork deals with monetary issues, let's look now at how the finances are coordinated for a training institute.

Financial/Accounting/Budgets/Funding

A training institute is a business. Like any business, funds must come from somewhere. The funding for most training institutes comes from student tuition, grants, or in-kind services from a parent agency. Any surplus funds are usually used for capital and training equipment improvements. The executive director is responsible for overseeing the finances of the institute. This section looks at how a training institute financially exists and plans its programs around the available funding sources.

BUDGET

An institute functions according to its budget. A budget consists of more than just dollar amounts. To arrive at a yearly budget, planning and preparation are required. Training program schedules, personnel costs, training equipment purchases and refurbishment, capital improvements, training supplies, office equipment, and office supplies are some of the categories in a typical budget. Many of these items require extensive planning, planning that is not financial in nature. Take, for instance, the training program schedule. The dollar amount for this item is based on the number of training programs that are projected for a year. Training surveys and other educational research studies are needed to come up with the number of training programs. Only then are course fees and the overall training budget determined.

The student tuition fee for a training program reflects the overall training institute costs. How a training institute is established—for example, separate corporation or a part of a larger parent organization—affects how the use of in-kind services is recognized. Copying costs, facility usage, and even personnel resources are potential sources of in-kind services. The in-kind services a training institute uses usually translate to a reduction in program costs and reduce the student's tuition fee. Any in-kind services should be identified and the dollar amount attached to these services in the budget. An executive director must know the total operating costs, and these include the in-kind services.

FUNDING

Student tuition is usually considered a primary source of funding for a training institute, but it is not the only source. Depending on how a training institute is affiliated—for example, with a college, community college, or vocational-technical school—federal and/or state funding for training may exist.

Depending on a state's funding of emergency service training, state grants may also be available. Training equipment, facility rental fees, textbooks, reproduction costs, course coordination costs, and instructor fees can be reimbursed through these state grants. Usually these grants are paid on a reimbursement basis. This means that a training institute is reimbursed only for the funds that the institute actually uses. The institute must front the initial expenditures and wait for the reimbursement. Although the training institute eventually gets its money, it does create a cash-flow problem for many training institutes.

For some institutes, even county governments or municipalities provide funding. These local funding sources are usually used to support the training of local emergency personnel. One way these local funds are used is to defer the full tuition fee for emergency personnel attending the training programs. Another alternative is to use the local funds to help support the operation of the training institute.

An executive director has key decisions to make regarding what funding options are appropriate for the training institute. Balancing in-kind resources with federal, state, and local funding resources and then arriving at a student tuition fee are not easy tasks. Once the budget is created, the executive director's task is to stay within the budget, the subject of the next section.

FINANCIAL MANAGEMENT AND ACCOUNTING

Regardless of the size of a training institute, sound financial management must be in place. Efficient financial planning, accounting, and payroll are critical financial areas. An institute should base its accounting system on generally accepted accounting principles and conduct a yearly audit. In addition, monthly financial statements need to be reviewed by the institute's administration. The continuation of a training institute is dependent upon the efficient management of the financial resources.

The concepts surrounding financial issues are foreign to most instructors. An everyday instructor rarely gets involved with the financial management of a training institute. Only when reimbursement checks are late will instructors have any interest in the finances of the training institute. Even then, all they really want to know is when they are going to be paid.

So why is all this financial stuff being mentioned? No, this is not an accounting lesson—it is an awareness discussion. Instructors should realize that there is a lot more to operating a training institute than just teaching students. If tuition fees and other funding cannot cover the institute expenses, instructors may see training programs being canceled and the training institute reducing instructional staff. This is often the consequence of poor financial management. The institute's administration must plan yearly budgets and training schedules to fit the anticipated capital. Similar to the educational concept of planning, presenting, and evaluating, a training administrator must plan annual budgets, pay out expenses, and audit the effectiveness of the institute's financial management. Having a balanced financial report while providing quality training programming is the chief goal for a training institute.

A factor that affects the finances and quantity of training is how a training institute advertises its programs.

Program Advertisement

Just because an institute budget outlines specific types of training programs, that does not mean that all of them will run. If the population— for example, the prospective students for a training program—is not aware of the training program, it is doubtful that the program will be run (Figure 15-5). This section looks at ways emergency service training programs can be advertised.

Aside from the grapevine network, there are other methods for a training institute to advertise emergency-service training programs. Each one has a price tag attached to it. Many training institutes cannot afford some of the advertising ideas that are about to be identified. Not having an ef-

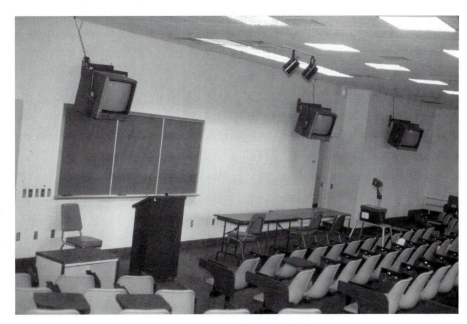

Figure 15-5
A training institute
can have the best of
facilities available,
but if the seats aren't
filled, no one can use
the facility.

fective advertising campaign can affect the number of students who attend a training program. The prices that are listed for each method are ballpark estimates. An institute's demographics (e.g., urban versus rural) often impact advertising costs.

BROCHURE/BULK MAIL

A front-line advertising approach used by many institutes is a program brochure. The brochure is usually a single-sheet flyer that lists the type of training program, times, dates, location, and the primary instructor. The tuition fee and registration section are usually included in a separate area of the brochure. These brochures are sent directly to individual students and emergency-service agencies. Using special bulk postal rates, a 1,000-piece mailing (including brochure development, copying costs, assembly time, and postage costs) can range from $450 to $700. Professionally printed brochures are more appealing but cost more toward the higher end of the range. Copier-machine copies tend to be less expensive but are less professional looking than the printed brochures.

PROGRAM CATALOG

This is a step up from the basic program brochure. Often a training institute will advertise each semester's programs. All training programs that are being offered are listed in the catalog. Detailed descriptions of each program are included in the catalog. There is a significant difference in the cost of a catalog versus that of a brochure. A mailing of 1,000 catalogs will run between $700 and $1,500. Again, copier-machine copies are less professional appearing than professionally printed brochures.

NEWSPAPER AND TRAINING MAGAZINES

Before leaping to this form of advertising, some serious research and planning must occur. The number one consideration is, "Who is the audience?" If the emergency training program is designed for recruiting the general public, then advertising in a local newspaper may be appropriate. But if the population for the training program is a specific group of emergency service personnel, newspaper advertising may not be a wise decision. Trade journals are probably the advertising location for specific-population-oriented training programs. So before any consideration can be made to use print media, an institute must define the target audience.

An audiovisual aid concept is often used in developing newspaper ads. That concept is to keep the material simple and to the point. A lot of written text will be ignored by most readers. Keep the written text to a minimum. It is important to hit the major ideas like type of course, times, dates, and locations. Identify a contact phone number and/or address for additional training program information.

The size of the ad will be affected by how much an institute is willing to pay. Depending on the newspaper company, the cost per column inch is a variable figure. Take, for instance, a two-column-wide by 6-inch-long ad (12 column inches), which is about a 4-inch by 6-inch size ad. A metropolitan newspaper may charge $700 and up for this size retail ad. A suburban newspaper, for the same ad, may charge $200 to $400. Rural newspaper costs are even less. Classified advertisements tend to be cheaper than retail advertising. The impact of the advertisement is often lost if it appears with multiple other ads in a similar format. Classified ads can usually be set only in boldface or underlined, and any creativity is lost when an ad appears in this section. Again, it goes back to who the audience is and what geographical area the students are being drawn from. These questions impact whether or not to use a newspaper advertising campaign.

Trade journals are a vital resource for advertising specific training programs. For specific audiences—for example, firefighters, high-angle rescue personnel, aeromedical personnel, or EMS managers—these trade journals can deliver a training institute's advertisement to the target audience. Per-column-inch costs are comparable to metropolitan newspaper costs. A trade journal that has a large circulation will have a higher per-column-inch fee than a trade journal with a small circulation. Because of the target audience, even though trade journals are more expensive than newspaper advertising, they may be a better option for training institutes.

RADIO ADVERTISING

Many prospective students tune into commercial radio stations on their way to and from work. Even at work, many prospective students are listening to commercial radio programs. Both AM and FM radio stations have an appreciable listening audience. Advertising on the radio is one way to attract the general public to a training program. The question to ask here is, Is the general public the target audience, or is the audience a specific emergency service audience? If the audience is the general public, then radio advertising is probably a reasonable alternative. However, if the training program is only for a specific group of emergency-service personnel and that group of personnel is rather small, then radio advertising probably is not the best method of advertising.

Aside from defining the audience, there are other significant factors involved in radio advertising. Like newspapers, the type of radio station location (e.g., large city versus small town), the station's listening audience, and even the radio station's format (e.g., country, soft rock, classical, top 40) are determinants that should be considered. These determinants also are used to set the costs involved in radio advertising. A 30-second radio spot in a large-city market costs several thousand dollars; the same ad broadcast in a smaller radio station market could run all week long for a thousand dollars. Radio ads may reach more people than newspapers, according to current market research. Depending upon the size of a training institute's advertising budget, one radio ad could spend the yearly budget allocation for many training institutes. As with any advertising option, a training institute must select those that fit the audience and stay within the budget.

CABLE TV AND COMMERCIAL TV

Most cities, suburban areas, and small communities have cable TV. Often these cable television agencies have a channel set aside for community-oriented advertising. These advertising channels offer reasonable rates for short messages. The messages usually last for 15 or 30 seconds.

Commercial TV is another option. However, the costs are significantly higher than the cable TV option. An actual videotaped advertisement would need to be developed. These development costs, plus the cost of 30 seconds of air time, make commercial TV a limited option for most training institutes.

ADVERTISING SUMMARY

Training institutes need to advertise the training programs that they are conducting. Most institutes use several advertising options to get the message out to their target audience. For most training institutes, there is not a lot of money set aside for advertising. A training institute must select advertising options that will maximize the available funding. Advertising is necessary to fill classrooms with students. Filling classes with qualified students is one of the missions for a training institute. Once in the classroom, the institute must assure that the students get a quality education. Besides providing advertising and quality education, there are added features that make a training program a special learning experience. These added features are discussed next.

Extra Perks in a Course

There is much more to a training program than just good instructors, sound educational training facilities, and effective program administration. To make a program a special learning experience often takes a variety of extra features. What perks are being discussed? These are features that make the difference between a good program and a great program. The following list identifies extra features that make a program a special experience:

- Personalized notebook and pencils
- Carpeted training rooms for practice sessions that require students to practice skills on the floor
- Access to coffee and/or soft drinks during break sessions
- For special weekend sessions, refreshments and lunches for the students
- Adequate parking within a reasonable distance to the training facility

Additional items could be included, but this list provides a sampling of the types of extras that make a program unique. Any extras that an instructor or training institute can include will enhance a training program. Making a program special is an extra bonus for students. These extras make an average program become a great program. But just having these extras does not make a quality learning experience. A lot more than these extras are needed. Chapter 11 looked extensively at how to evaluate a training program's quality. The next section reviews the concepts of quality assurance for a training institute.

Quality Improvement for Training Institutes

Quality programming is a responsibility of the entire institute. Chapter 11 identified the need to develop institute objectives and assessment mechanisms to assess a program's quality. Instructors and program administrators jointly develop these quality assurance mechanisms. Quality assurance issues should be identified during a program instead of being identified after a program ends (Figure 15-6). Both positive and weak areas need to be

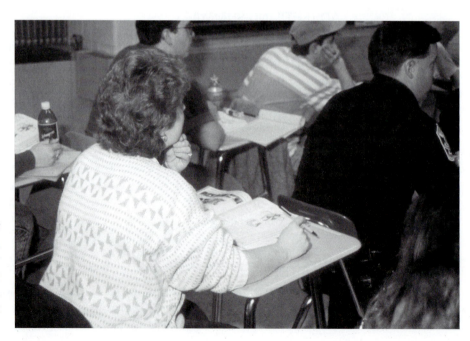

Figure 15-6
Quality education doesn't happen by accident. A training institute must work at providing the best training possible.

identified. Too often, only poor qualities of a training program are highlighted. Highlighting only poor qualities is not an objective assessment of a training program. In an effective quality assurance program, both good and poor aspects of a program are highlighted.

Assessing the quality of a training program is a primary role of either the training administrator and/or executive director. Instructors and course coordinators are usually too involved with the logistics and instruction of a training program to objectively assess the quality assurance aspects. The person who does the quality assurance assessment needs to be objective. Not being actively involved in a program becomes a prerequisite for a person conducting the assessment. Only with objective information will a program be fairly assessed. Training institutes and instructors want to provide the best training possible. Assessing the quality of a program helps a training institute do just that.

In many states, training institutes must comply with a set of minimum performance standards. The institute must become accredited to continue offering training programs. The next section looks at how a training institute becomes accredited.

Training Institute Accreditation

Not only do training institutes need to assess their program's quality, often they must comply with standards established by a state or an independent agency. Depending on the state where a training institute is located, there may be mandatory standards that a training institute must meet (Figure 15-7).

Accreditation standards usually set performance and facility requirements that a training institute must meet. If a training site lacks critical components, the institute may not be allowed to conduct programs until

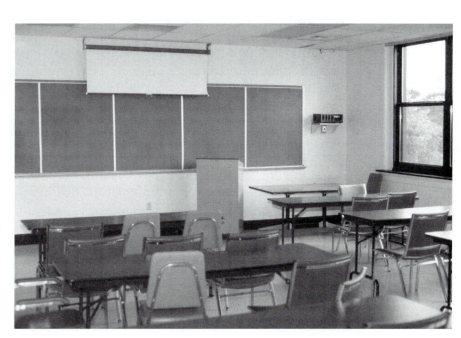

Figure 15-7
The accreditation process not only looks at classrooms, but it examines the entire training institute.

the components are corrected. Components that are frequently reviewed during an accreditation include

Training Facilities
—Room size compared with number of students
—Room free of noise
—Adequate lighting in the rooms
—AV aids in rooms
—Access to rest rooms
—Facility safety

Training Equipment
—Adequate quantities for number of students being trained
—Routine maintenance schedule and maintenance records
—Meets minimum types of equipment identified by accreditation

Faculty
—Identification of primary and secondary instructors
—Review of instructor's performance on a regular basis
—Identify clinical and field preceptors

Administration
—Identification of personnel for the institute
—Disclosure of annual records for student enrollment, budgets, pass/fail ratios, quality assurance records, and related performance documentation

This is a partial listing of issues that are considered during an accreditation inspection. Once an institute receives accreditation, the accreditation is usually good for two or three years. This accreditation certification means that at the time an institute was inspected, it met the minimum standards established by the accrediting agency.[2]

Aside from state agencies issuing accreditations to training institutes, independent groups often review institutes. These independent groups usually have more stringent standards for institutes to meet. Attaining these types of accreditations shows that a training institute has exceeded standards beyond the minimum and has set high levels of excellence for the education of its students.

Whether or not the accreditation is mandatory, most training institutes are accountable to someone. Instructors should realize that their performance plays a part in the accreditation of an institute. Instructors are the front line for assuring quality education. Accrediting agencies frequently review the performance of instructors during their visits. Instructors should try to conduct their presentations as if no one were monitoring them, although this is hard to do. Still, the more relaxed and "normal" a class session, the better the ratings will be for the instructor. Even if the overhead projector malfunctions, and there are too few handouts for the stu-

---

[2]Pennsylvania Department of Health Training Institute Accreditation Policies (Harrisburg, Penn.: 1999).

dents, and the wrong quiz has been copied, all are events that challenge an instructor. A reviewer will be interested to see how an instructor copes with these events. When a course coordinator says, "There are some reviewers coming to see your session," do not become a nervous wreck. Keep calm and teach the class as if they were not there. Reviewing instructors is a part of the accreditation process. It is only one component of the accreditation process, so instructors should not feel that the entire institute's accreditation is resting on their performance. If an institute is going to fail an inspection, there will be more reasons than a projector failing to operate!

Summary

The intent of this chapter is to make instructors aware that they are one piece in the training puzzle. The umbrella of training administration covers a wide variety of individuals. A training program does not just appear. Only through a lot of people behind the scenes, working together, does a training program become a quality learning experience for students.

Providing quality education is what this entire book has addressed. Quality education starts with each person having a desire to do the best job. Instructors are the front-line personnel. Students usually see only their instructors and course coordinator. The reputation of a training institute is placed into the hands of its instructors. Successful instructors mean successful programs in most cases. Instructors need a logistical network to be the best they can be. An institute's administration is the logistical network for an instructor. A breakdown in the network will affect both the instructor and the students. But in the end, everyone will be affected by someone's poor performance: The instructor, the course coordinator, the administrators, the entire institute, and especially the students. Effective program administration, combined with innovative and dynamic instructors, is a recipe for a quality educational experience.

Quality educational experiences are what students deserve. If emergency service personnel are to be expected to deliver the best care or service possible, they must have a quality education. That is the ultimate mission for everyone who instructs emergency service training programs.

Index